CHASING
BEAUTY

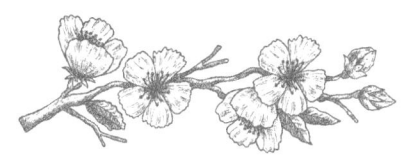

CHASING
BEAUTY

The Art, Science, and Business of Aesthetics

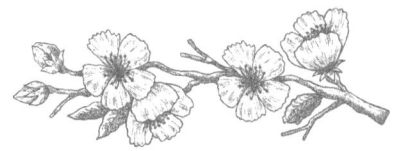

Lycia Thornburg MD, FAAD

Chasing Beauty: The Art, Science, and Business of Aesthetics
Copyright ©2025 Lycia Thornburg

All rights reserved. No portion of this book may be reproduced in any form, by any means, electronic or mechanical, including photocopying, recording, or by any information storage and retrieval system, without permission in writing from the publisher.

First Edition
Printed in the United States of America.

Cover design by Jake Clark, Pithy Wordsmithery
Interior design by Sue Murray, Pithy Wordsmithery
Copy Editing by Nils Kuehn, Pithy Wordsmithery
Proofreading by Katharine Dvorak and Scott Morrow, Pithy Wordsmithery

ISBN: 979-8-9924157-0-4 (Paperback)
ISBN: 979-8-9924157-1-1 (Ebook)
ISBN: 979-8-9924157-2-8 (Hardback)

Lycia Thornburg
https://www.lyciathornburgmd.com
lct@rap.midco.net

Library of Congress Control Number: 2025901345

Praise

"This book is a must-read for anybody who is thinking about dipping their toe into the pool of aesthetic dermatology."
—Jeanine Downie, MD, FAAD

"Chasing Beauty translates the latest dermatological research into practical, easy-to-follow steps. Dr. Thornburg's skill in blending scientific breakthroughs with real-world advice makes this book an essential tool for anyone."
—Emerald L. Christopher, PhD

"This book contains secrets about the field of aesthetics. Dr. Thornburg reveals these so eloquently and non-judgmentally that you owe it to yourself to invest in reading this book. If you're a consumer, this will help you sift through the hype of a prospective practitioner and choose one based on relevant criteria. If you're a practitioner, you will want to hear the other side of the territorial conversation. A must-read!"
—Leslie Fletcher, MSN, AGNP-BC

"Dr. Thornburg masterfully combines medical expertise with a holistic approach to beauty, making this book essential for anyone committed to lasting skin health."
—Kathleen O'Brien, PA-C

"This is a great read for anyone hoping to increase patient satisfaction in the crowded world of aesthetic dermatology."
—Jacqueline M. Calkin, MD, FAAD

"Chasing Beauty highlights the essential link between community and collaboration, showing how we can uplift one another regardless of background. By focusing on patient care through empathy, we create a supportive environment that benefits everyone. A transformative read that inspires deeper connections."
—Trevor Larsen, RN

"Dr. Thornburg has masterfully infused her own personality and wisdom into Chasing Beauty. It is well written, easy to read, and sure to become a landmark publication in the field."
—Dr. Nicholas Howland, MD, FACS

Dedication

For my husband and girls.

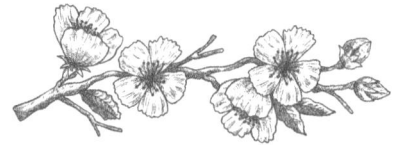

Table of Contents

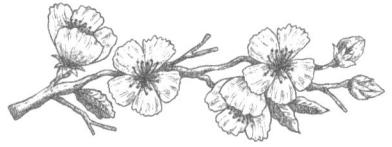

Preface ix
Introduction xv

Chapter 1: Chasing Beauty... 1
Chapter 2: The Wild West.. 10
Chapter 3: A New Approach 20
Chapter 4: Vitamins and Nutrition 29
Chapter 5: Sun Protection.. 41
Chapter 6: Step Up Your Skincare Routine 51
Chapter 7: Light and Lasers 69
Chapter 8: Botox 83
Chapter 9: Filler 100
Chapter 10: The Skinny on Weight-Loss Treatments 117
Chapter 11: Radiofrequency 130
Chapter 12: Microneedling, Plasma-Rich Protein, and Exosomes . 134
Chapter 13: Putting It All Together 147

Quick Guide for Aesthetic Treatments, by Age........................... 161
Quick Guide for Spotting Cancer 168
Acknowledgments 173
About the Author 175
Endnotes 177

Preface

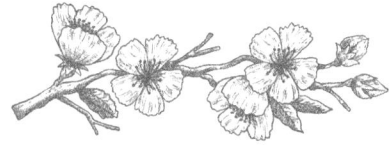

I walk toward the podium, blinded by the spotlights. Carefully navigating the path, I take a deep breath and hope I don't forget what I want to say. As I look out into the audience, I see the leaders in our community. Successful entrepreneurs, executives, doctors, philanthropists. Passionate, highly intelligent people who get things done. Diamonds sparkle on perfectly manicured fingers, and people smile up at me politely between bites of delicious food prepared by a brilliant chef. This is the kind of room that would have intimidated me when I was younger. But today, I am the driving force that brought everyone together.

Coming from a middle-class family in Wisconsin, it was hard for me to picture the kind of life I have now. I went to UW–Madison on a scholarship. I felt a pull toward the medical field, so I decided that I would declare pre-med as my major. But when I met with my guidance counselor, he tried to dissuade me by telling me that the *men* who get into that program usually have higher GPAs. I wasn't sure what to be insulted about more: the fact that he didn't think women should pursue medicine or that after one year of school, he didn't think I had the potential to graduate with a high GPA. That got to me. For a while, I wondered if perhaps I wasn't cut out for becoming a doctor. But ultimately, I decided to go for it anyway. I transferred to the University of Wyoming and found a biology lab that inspired me on a daily basis to become a doctor. I'm thankful that I believed in myself, had parents who encouraged me, and made the decision to pursue medicine even though certain people around me thought it was a long shot.

In med school, among the wide variety of specialties we explored, I enjoyed pediatrics, adult medicine, surgery, and clinic. But I found

Preface

myself most drawn toward dermatology. I'd had eczema when I was young, so the doctor I saw the most growing up was my dermatologist—in fact, I thought everyone had a dermatologist. Dermatology was one of the only fields that allowed all these aspects of medicine to be tied to one specialty. It was one of the best decisions I ever made, and I can truly say that I've found my calling.

In my first years of practicing, I met countless patients who were dealing with skin complications that could have been prevented if they'd had better protection from the sun. Many of them had spent their childhoods playing outside in the hot South Dakota summers and were just learning about the importance of sunscreen. They didn't know that sun exposure damages skin-cell DNA, and the younger you are when sun damage occurs, the more problems it can cause. Most could remember having at least a few sunburns at a young age.

Now, decades later, they were getting malignant melanoma. I did my best to cut out cancerous tissue and keep it from spreading and becoming fatal. Sometimes, patients went on to live healthy, full lives. Other times, there was only so much we could do.

I couldn't help but fixate on how so much of this hardship and suffering was preventable. I racked my brain on what I could do to make a difference. After many, many hours worrying about the patients I was currently treating, it dawned on me that the solution was to have helped them earlier in life.

Children's skin is more sensitive and delicate than that of adults, making it more susceptible to sunburn and damage from UV radiation. Early sunburns can significantly increase the risk of developing skin cancer, including melanoma, later in life. Protecting children's skin from an early age helps reduce their lifetime risk of skin cancer.

As a mother of young girls, I know how hard it is to keep kids out of the sun. They want to run free outside, and parents want that for their kids too. They need to burn off energy or else they turn into little terrors. There's no good way around the need to go outside for fresh air and exercise a couple times a day. But with the great outdoors comes dangerous sun exposure. I experienced this with my kids on a daily basis. No matter where we went, the sun always seemed to be beating down right on top of us. I found myself exhausted by constantly

Preface

pinning down squirming children and applying sunscreen, reapplying more sunscreen, and forcing their little hats back on their heads.

South Dakota isn't known for warm weather, but our summers are scorchers. In the Black Hills, we're at elevation, which makes the sun more powerful than in many other parts of the country. You can feel this intensity outside on playgrounds and soccer fields and even just walking down the street. I was always looking for a respite, a small patch of shade to catch my breath and give my kids' skin a break.

This is how I got the idea to start my nonprofit organization, Made for Shade. The idea was simple: create an option for people—especially children—to get out of the sun without having to go indoors. This could be done by planting more trees, building permanent shade structures in parks, and having pop-up tents at outdoor events.

As a dermatologist, I know that a little shade goes a long way. For example, kids often play on the same playground equipment at recess, two times a day, five days a week. An umbrella shade over the structure could provide kids around five hours of sun protection a week—for years—which could be the difference in preventing deadly skin cancer.

Once my mission was clear, I began working hard to build the organization that would make it happen. Eighteen years later, looking out into the audience, I feel a chill go up my spine.

The organization has transformed. I have transformed. And so has my family. I used to need a babysitter to stay home with my kids during the annual gala. Now, my oldest is chatting with our largest sponsors and sipping a glass of wine.

The first few years, it was a struggle to get funding for projects and corporate sponsors. Slowly, we gained support locally with construction donations to install our structures. We were blessed to partner with Riddle's, a large diamond retail chain that donated many beautiful pieces of jewelry for us to auction off at our events. Over time, we received backing from industry-leading organizations in the form of matching grants from Neutrogena and repeated support from Allergan, the maker of Botox. After many years of hard work, I'm proud to declare that we raised over $325,000 for 78 projects. It took time, but we are now well known in our community—and also outside of it.

Preface

A key factor that has helped Made for Shade grow is the societal shift in how people think about skincare. Aesthetic dermatology has been experiencing a renaissance. People always yearn to look young and beautiful, and with recent advances in technology, numerous treatment modalities and products are being developed to treat the exact areas people want to target. Today, skincare is *en vogue*.

The world has woken up to the importance of safeguarding one's skin against cancer, and many people are now just as focused on keeping their skin looking young and beautiful. The rise in aesthetic dermatology has completely changed the way we think about skin. With advances in technology, we have numerous treatment modalities and products to enhance the exact areas people want to target. I have always been fascinated by the science behind this, and I embrace it for my patients. In addition to continuing to practice general dermatology, my office currently has more than $1 million worth of aesthetics machines.

The world has woken up to the importance of safeguarding one's skin against cancer, and many people are now just as focused on keeping their skin looking young and beautiful.

Despite how much my patients love the services we offer, I've gotten a significant amount of pushback for how I've chosen to expand my practice. I've learned firsthand that when doctors shift to aesthetics, their peers often think it's selling out—as though elective treatments aren't real medicine and the people who perform them aren't real doctors. As more and more patients came to me for filler, laser treatment, and Botox, I catch more and more side-eye from some doctors in my community.

Meanwhile, as medical doctors opt out of participating in the fastest-growing segment of healthcare, the industry is experiencing serious growing pains. With any new industry, there are problems. Certain necessary regulations aren't in place, and things go wrong without proper safety protocols.

With more interest in skincare, the amount of advice available online—some of it good, most of it bad—has become staggering. It's frightening to me how many people with huge followings on social media are dispensing false and dangerous information regarding skincare.

Preface

I decided to write this book because I see a great need for practitioners in the industry to level up their knowledge and skills and take a more patient-centered approach. With collaboration, we can rise together for the benefit of our patients. Whether you have a role in the aesthetics space or are simply intrigued by the mysteries of new treatment modalities, I hope you find it to be an indispensable guide.

Introduction

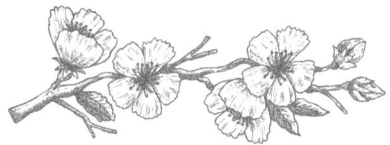

To experience another person is to hear their voice, listen to their perspective, and get a window into their soul. But it's also looking in their eyes, seeing their smile, and sometimes touching their skin.

We say it's what's on the inside that matters, but the reality is that the inside is trapped under the outside. The whole person is the inside *and* the outside. This is an uncomfortable truth because there are many aspects of our skin envelopes that we cannot fully control. When we feel different on the inside than how we look on the outside, it can cause a painful dissonance.

Humans are social creatures. We want to be loved and accepted. Throughout history, people have been intentional about improving their outward appearance using whatever methods were within their span of control. From ancient Egyptians using kohl to line their eyes to Europeans in the Middle Ages plucking their hairlines to achieve higher foreheads, people have always strived to meet societal standards of beauty.

Medicine and science have made leaps and bounds in the past several decades. There are now many options for products, treatments, and procedures that make a noticeable difference—especially when it comes to our faces. Being 50 years old today can look totally different than it has throughout human history. The demand for aesthetic services has skyrocketed, and the industry is expanding at a staggering pace. With the rapid evolution of technology, the quality of results is increasing while costs are decreasing, making services more accessible.

The global aesthetics market size was valued at $374 billion in 2023, is projected to grow to $393 billion in 2024, and could reach

Introduction

$758 billion by 2032, exhibiting a compound annual growth rate of 9.8 percent during the forecast period.[1]

Although the numbers clearly show both the demand for, and value of, these services, the medical industry largely eschews practices it deems to be elective and inconsequential to people's health.

I started practicing medicine in general dermatology, but I was always interested in the science behind aesthetic dermatology. When Botox first came out around 2003, I was graduating from my medical school residency at the University of Iowa, which is among the nation's top dermatology programs. One of the creators of Botox came to our campus to train us on this new neuromodulator.[2] Previously used to treat children with spastic limbs, it was now a way to help patients smooth out their wrinkles. I was fascinated.

Although it took over a decade for Botox to start really catching on, it was the spark that began the slow burn into the growth of the aesthetics space. Dermatology was no longer just about services that patients *needed*; it was also about services they *wanted*.

In the years that followed, we saw bovine collagen being used as filler to treat wrinkles, and then came the shift to hyaluronic acids. Voluma entered the market in 2016 and it became possible to make cheeks look much fuller with simple injections. After that, a new generation of lasers entered the market, allowing us to generate new collogen without ablating the skin like the old carbon dioxide (C_{O2}) lasers that would burn patients. Thanks to their functionality being controlled by computers, a few years ago, C_{O2} laser technology leveled up another notch, leading to significantly better safety and quality control.

Looking back, the transformation has been a total whirlwind. A lot has changed in the world since the early 2000s, and this is one of those industries that simply didn't use to exist. Being a part of the progress has been nothing if not exciting. I've always leaned into it, attending all the aesthetic dermatology training sessions and conferences I could fit into my busy physician's schedule. Over the years, my practice has consis-tently invested in new aesthetic dermatology machines, and I've seen an overwhelmingly positive response from patients. What's more, patients coming into the office more often for treatments has given additional opportunities to assess their skin. I can't tell you how many times I've

Introduction

noticed a weird mark or bump, biopsied it, and found cancer. Catching skin cancer early is a godsend for patients and incredibly rewarding for me as a doctor.

Today, about 60 percent of my patients come in for general dermatology and 40 percent come in for aesthetic services. Even though the majority of my work falls squarely in traditional medicine, I've gotten significant pushback and passive-aggressive commentary from other doctors about my decision to practice aesthetic dermatology. I've been told that I've turned the dermatology office into a spa. (This feedback was delivered in a way that made it clear it wasn't a compliment!) When I made the list of the best injectors in the nation, aesthetics-industry leaders and practitioners I knew around the country congratulated me, while some of the doctors I worked most closely with didn't say a word. On a personal level, though, I've never lost any sleep over this; it is the canary in the coal mine of a much larger problem.

As doctors and the medical community at large intentionally distance themselves from aesthetic practices, the industry is experiencing dangerous growing pains. As seen in virtually all emerging industries, innovation in aesthetics is outpacing regulation, and we find ourselves operating in the "Wild West." The glaring lack of formal oversight, laws, and safety measures is leaving both patients and practitioners increasingly vulnerable.

One of the most popular aesthetic treatments, injecting filler, is a real medical procedure with an implantable device. And whenever you implant something into the body, there are risks. Aside from potentially leading to infection, it can kill tissue, causing the skin to die and turn blue/black. Injecting near the eyes can also cause blindness—a catastrophic consequence for any patient.

Granted, there are remedies for treating some of these conditions. But after attending industry tradeshows and events and talking with a number of aesthetic practitioners, I've become acutely aware of how unprepared many practices are to treat adverse outcomes.

To treat dying tissue, the antidote must be mixed properly and injected quickly, and the medicine cannot be expired—something that happens easily when supplies aren't frequently used up. Since adequate amounts of the antidote cost $5,000 and are likely to be

Introduction

periodically thrown away over the years, many practitioners simply don't have it on hand.

To treat sudden blindness, you only have eight minutes to take action before it will become permanent. The treatment is another medical procedure, which should ideally be done by an ophthalmologist. Most med spas don't have this type of medical professional at their disposal in case of emergency.

Many patients don't understand these risks. Worse, many injectors don't either. Filler parties poolside in the Hamptons sound glamorous, and many practitioners and patients enjoy them, but what happens when something doesn't go as planned?

Having heard the horror stories of aesthetic medicine causing permanent injury, and understanding how easy it is to prevent these issues, I've made it my personal mission to help move the industry in a positive direction.

It's time for aesthetic practitioners, board-certified dermatologists and plastic surgeons, and doctors with a variety of focus areas to be proactive and level up their knowledge and skills.

In this book, I cover what practitioners need to know in order to improve their craft, serve patients better, and become much-needed partners in guiding the industry through its infancy stage, which will only create better and safer outcomes. Throughout, I include citations so you can refer to the full studies I highlight and learn more.

This book will also help patients better understand how the industry operates, the types of treatments available to them, and what they should keep in mind when considering aesthetic treatments.

The first few chapters set the scene for where we are today and where we're headed. From there, I cover the "low-hanging fruit" when it comes to looking our best, including vitamins, nutrition, and sun-protection solutions. It might not sound sexy, but these are the bases everyone should cover before they even consider doing any types of aesthetic treatments at a clinic or med spa. Next, I do a deep dive into the skincare products that actually work and why. I explain the proper steps for a daily skincare routine—at any budget.

Introduction

For aesthetics practitioners, you should make it your job to inform your patients of these kinds of simple things they can do on their own to make their skin as healthy as possible outside of treatments.

The second half of the book is dedicated to demystifying a variety of professional aesthetic services and treatment modalities, including the types of scenarios for which they are excellent options, how to best use them, and the pitfalls to avoid. I examine patients' perceptions of these services, the types of outcomes they can expect, and how the services fit into a full portfolio of aesthetic offerings from a practitioner.

At the end of the book, I tie it all together and explain how multiple types of treatments can be used together to get the best possible results. I also provide a quick guide for recognizing key signs of skin cancer. Knowing what to look for can help you catch it early and save your life.

Whether you are a seasoned professional with a role in the aesthetics space, just getting started in your profession, a patient receiving these treatments, or simply intrigued by the mysteries of new treatment modalities, this book is your indispensable guide. Let's go on a journey together where innovation meets responsibility and where beauty finds its rightful place in the realm of science.

Chapter 1

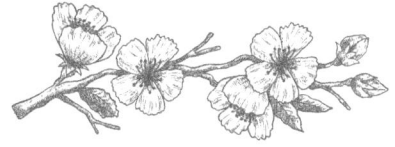

Chasing Beauty

It's a quiet, sunny morning, and a woman sits down to do her makeup. She has an important event this afternoon, and it's crucial that she looks her best. She didn't sleep well because her youngest child, a toddler, kept waking up throughout the night and needed to be rocked back to sleep. Now the woman has dark circles under her eyes. She searches through her cosmetics to find a product that can disguise how tired she feels.

Just the other day, her sister was teasing her for starting to look more and more like their mother. Although her comments weren't meant maliciously, they still stung. She knows that she's been looking older lately—a reality that leaves her with an unsettling feeling in the pit of her stomach. She used to turn heads walking down the street, but that now seems like a lifetime ago.

She notices that her skin *feels* older to the touch, whereas her children's skin is smooth, taut, and plump. Her toddler's chubby cheeks are almost bouncy when she pokes them! Reaching up to her own cheeks, the texture is totally different. It's almost like her skin is becoming too big for her.

She feels like wallowing in her misery, but she doesn't have time for that. One of her kids is sure to need something or start crying any minute. Working quickly, she applies a moisturizer, eye makeup, blush, and lip gloss. That will have to do for now. Her friends swear by a new beauty treatment they say takes years off their faces, but she will have to treat herself to that when she finds the time.

How did you picture the woman in this story? She could be any one of millions of women alive today, but I wrote this anecdote specifically thinking about an Egyptian woman living 3,000 years ago. Just like today, women in ancient Egypt wore makeup and used beauty products. Although mirrors didn't exist back then, people were able to check their appearance in reflection bowls or highly polished metal discs.[3] Ancient Egyptians were concerned about aging because youthfulness was the idealized norm, as it represented eternity.[4] With this in mind, they took the time and effort to look their best. Even the humblest of graves have consistently been found to contain at least a small supply of makeup.[5]

Despite so many things having changed in the past 3,000 years, the desire to look young and beautiful has withstood the test of time.

Despite so many things having changed in the past 3,000 years, the desire to look young and beautiful has withstood the test of time.

Although there is great variation when it comes to the beauty standards of various eras, societies, and places throughout history, I've found a common thread throughout my research: a woman's value has almost always been tied to her looks. This isn't to say that particularly attractive men don't have an advantage over other men, but it's generally been a much bigger advantage for women. Why is this? Well, men have typically been the ruling gender. They've held the power. They've made the decisions. Volumes of books could be written on this topic alone, but for our purposes here, I will keep it brief.

In early human societies, physical strength was a significant advantage for survival, particularly when it came to hunting and protection. Men, on average, have always had greater physical strength, which often positioned them in roles that were more highly valued in terms of power and status. Meanwhile, women's roles in childbearing and childrearing often limited their ability and desire to participate in activities outside the home. This division of labor entrenched gender roles and made it more challenging for women to make headway in leadership roles outside their own homes.

Further, many societies developed cultural and religious norms that justified and perpetuated male dominance. These norms were often codified into laws and practices that restricted women's rights and opportunities. For example, patriarchal religions and traditions often placed only men in positions of authority and decision-making.

On top of cultural and religious norms pigeonholing women at home, men have historically controlled economic resources, which translated into power. Ownership of land, wealth, and businesses often remained in the hands of men, giving them significant influence over societal structures and decision-making processes. Combine that with political power excluding women and unequal access to education and we have millennia upon millennia of women who have existed almost as second-class citizens while men held all the power.

What power do women have? Well, the two things that men can't take from them: their beauty and their ability to bear children. To be more specific on the type of beauty that has almost always been most valued, it's the youthful type that women possess during their childbearing years. The fertile kind of beauty.

Beautiful young women in their fertile era have been able to elevate their status and power by attracting better suitors. For women, better looks have historically meant more options for a partner, greater financial security, and a better shot at happiness. It's a harsh truth.

Luckily, times are changing. In 1920, women in every state were granted the right to vote, which was a crucial step in shifting the power structure in the United States. More women are now seeking higher education than men. Heck, we can even get credit cards without a male relative cosigning for us (something that wasn't possible until 1974).[6] Women still don't typically earn as much as men do—for a number of reasons—but it's no longer impossible to support ourselves financially without a husband.

With the power balance shifting in favor of women, where does this leave the ancient tradition of chasing beauty? Is it simply out of habit? Or is there something deeper?

No matter how uncomfortable this might be for all of us to admit, there is still an inherent advantage that comes with being attractive. This is often called *pretty privilege*. Research has shown that people who are considered to be physically attractive tend to be more well liked or popular. This often makes life a bit easier from adolescence onward. There are career advantages as well. Studies suggest that conventionally attractive people have an advantage in hiring decisions, promotions, and salary, and they earn 10 to 15 percent more money to do the same jobs as those that are considered unattractive or "homely."[7]

On top of this, the advantages associated with pretty privilege can contribute to higher self-esteem and confidence—traits that serve a person well in life in myriad ways. Oh, and to go back to finding a partner, attractiveness obviously still plays a significant role in dating opportunities, with good-looking people being more sought after and having more options themselves. With all this in mind, being good looking seems to create a virtuous cycle.

Is this fair? Absolutely not. Does it exemplify a whole host of serious problems we could discuss at length, such as bias, "shallowness," and other societal shortcomings? Without a doubt. Countless books and research studies examine these topics. But for our purposes here, I will keep it simple: people—especially women—want to look attractive because it improves their opportunities in a variety of life's many facets, and even more importantly, because it makes them feel better about themselves.

That's why women continue chasing beauty even though we can make our own money and our own decisions and we don't need anyone to support us financially.

When I started as a dermatologist over 20 years ago, I was driven by the desire to help people stay healthy. Many of my patients have had life-threatening conditions, such as malignant melanoma, non-melanoma skin cancers, and autoimmune disease diagnosed through skin findings. More often, I've seen patients with skin conditions that aren't life threatening but impact their quality of life, whether it's from physical discomfort or an unusual appearance that makes them feel self-conscious or embarrassed. I learned early on that caring for patients means looking after them both physically and emotionally. When I could make an unsightly rash disappear, patients would overflow with gratitude—often even more so than the patients whose lives I actually saved (thanks to their yearly skin checks!). This reality has really stuck with me over the years.

People are acutely aware of how they feel about their appearance, and despite caring about their health, they don't always have the ability to gauge it.

Establishing guardrails

Without guardrails, the aesthetics industry has the power to create many negative outcomes. It's essential that we understand what's at stake and what we can do to help guide the industry in as healthy a direction as possible.

Champion age-appropriate marketing: Anti-aging used to be a thing people started thinking about in their 30s, 40s, or 50s. These days, teenagers and people in their 20s are getting treatments—not to mention all the kids and pre-teens graduating from toys to beauty products!

Oftentimes, these young people are interested in skincare products and treatments that aren't appropriate for their skin. Constantly applying products such as retinol, vitamin C, or hyaluronic acid to young, healthy skin can cause damage because the skin hasn't reached maturity yet. The same is true for harsh exfoliators, laser treatments, and peels. Getting filler on skin that's already tight can potentially stretch the skin.

But most young people don't know this because it's not what they hear in the media or online. According to a 2024 study, more than 56 percent of Gen Z turns to TikTok as a source for health and wellness information, and one in three use social media as their main source of health knowledge.[8] And if you've looked on social media recently, you've probably noticed that there are a lot of beauty influencers out there. Most of them aren't doctors, healthcare professionals, or even aesthetics professionals. Instead, they're kids and young people with pretty faces who have mastered what it takes to get social engagement. And who can blame them when society has influenced them into focusing on everlasting youth?

As adults, we have the responsibility of encouraging kids to be kids. Young people shouldn't be worrying about what they look like—and they certainly shouldn't be losing any sleep over aging. Let's work together to keep the industry marketing age appropriate and to weed out patients that are too young for our services.

Embrace natural features: With modern aesthetic treatments today, it's possible to dramatically alter a person's natural features. We can create higher cheekbones, change the shape of eyes and eyelids, make lips plump and pouty. We can reshape jawlines, regrow hair, make noses that have a cute little ski slope. And that's just on the face! When it comes to the body, we can drastically alter a person's shape, whether it's making them thinner or thicker. But just because it's possible to make these changes doesn't mean we should.

Dr. Emerald Christopher, adjunct lecturer at Georgetown University, has done considerable research on women's and gender studies, with an emphasis on marginalized women. She's noticed that the physical blueprint held up by society as the ideal has shifted over the years to align with certain traits that often come naturally to women of color. For example, she cites Kylie Jenner for her appropriation of thicker lips. Jenner spurred a movement in which women and girls became obsessed with achieving a lip shape that did not come naturally from their genetics.

The emphasis on achieving a look that doesn't naturally align with one's genetics can create a disconnect between appearance and one's cultural identity. It promotes a homogenized beauty ideal that overlooks the diversity of natural beauty across different cultures and ethnicities.

Further, Christopher points out that there's a double standard when features that were once ridiculed or devalued when associated with people of color suddenly become desirable when adopted by white celebrities or influencers. This dynamic reinforces existing racial and cultural hierarchies, wherein the dominant culture can pick and choose elements from marginalized cultures without facing the same scrutiny or consequences.

In the interviews I conducted for this book, my interviewees mentioned the Kardashians or Jenners almost every single time. They have certainly had an oversized impact in shaping modern beauty standards and also shown the world how it's possible to dramatically alter one's appearance through aesthetic treatments.

Patients will always come to us and ask for treatments to change their natural features. Instead of simply giving them what they want without any questions asked, I believe that we, as practitioners, have a responsibility to help them celebrate a wide range of natural beauty standards by encouraging the enhancement of their natural features instead of championing dramatic transformations.

Don't support obsession or addiction: More is not always more. We've all seen people who are addicted to beauty services, whether it's on TV, at the supermarket, or walking into a dermatologist's office. They look in the mirror and see flaws that no one else sees, so they spend outlandish amounts of money and time on enhancements. Some of these treatments only make marginal changes, which, after so many appointments, is probably a good thing. For others, things can go south quickly. Depending on the types of services they get and the level of quality they receive, they can end up looking fake, their features garish.

When patients don't know when to stop, practitioners need to help them. It should not be capitalism without care.

Additionally, as aesthetic practitioners, we need to be careful when it comes to our own treatments. With all the tools, supplies, and experts at our disposal, it's easy to do a little lasering here and a little filler there. And then a little more and a little more. It's important to keep a close eye on ourselves and know when enough is enough. There are a number of health implications from overdoing certain types of treatments, but the main concern I usually see is mental. It's not ideal to live in a world where we're always thinking about how life would be better if we looked just a little younger. Let's be kind to ourselves.

Make treatments accessible: As more and more people choose to have treatments, the bar for beauty standards only continues to be raised—and it's happening at lightning speed. Unfortunately, aesthetic treatments, such as fillers, laser treatments, fat freezing, and body-contouring procedures, are often expensive. The high cost makes these treatments accessible primarily to those with disposable income. Wealthier individuals can afford regular maintenance treatments, whereas those with fewer resources may be unable to access these services at all.

In societies where appearance plays a significant role in social and professional opportunities, access to aesthetic treatments can enhance a person's attractiveness, potentially influencing their perceived competence, confidence, and even job prospects. This creates a situation where those who can afford these treatments gain a competitive advantage, further widening the gap between rich and poor. In this way, access to aesthetic treatments could contribute to broader social inequalities, where appearance increasingly becomes a marker of wealth and privilege. This can perpetuate a cycle wherein the rich continue to enhance their social capital through appearance while the poor are further marginalized.

With this in mind, all players in the aesthetics industry need to think about how important it is to keep treatments as accessible as possible. We all need to earn a living, but we don't need to price gouge. This is true for drug makers, suppliers, manufactures, trainers, and practitioners alike.

Our call to action

As aesthetic practitioners, we find ourselves in a complex situation. People have always chased beauty, and that's unlikely to change in the future. However, we are now equipped like never before to help people achieve the results they dream of. This is a pivotal, exciting time in history. We want to help people feel their best. But at the same time, we must be conscious of the impacts we have in this role.

After I started leaning into aesthetic practices, I quickly saw the power that it has. Yes, it makes people look younger. But the real power is in transforming the way people feel about themselves. With a few pokes of the needle, it's like taking 5 to 10 years off someone's mentality. I began seeing the way women hold their heads higher. They stand up straighter and take up more space. They tell me about going for that promotion they've been wanting, or finally telling their partner that he'd better shape up or else. It helps women find the confidence they deserve, and because of that, they are leveling up their lives. I am thrilled and honored to play even the smallest role in these outcomes.

As we move forward in the industry, I encourage everyone to focus on the do-good component of aesthetics. By pairing this notion with the do-no-harm component of medicine, we can truly help the industry move forward in a positive direction.

Chapter 2

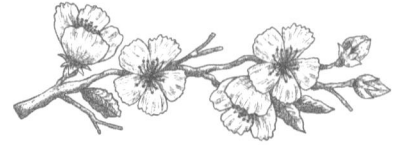

The Wild West

Whenever new industries emerge, there is always a lack of proper regulation because people don't understand exactly what's needed. Standards haven't been set, and there's no one to answer to when outcomes are subpar. Everything starts out as the Wild West. Individuals and companies operate however they see fit, and we watch it unfold in real time.

When social media platforms first gained traction, they operated with little oversight concerning privacy and data protection. Unauthorized data harvesting ran rampant, and data was misused in ways that were detrimental. In the 2010s, private companies such as Cambridge Analytica were able to strategically use personal information they'd harvested from 87 million Facebook users without their consent.[9] This data was then used to spread fake news online and influence public opinion in the 2016 US presidential election.[10]

When ride-sharing services entered the market, they operated in many areas without traditional taxi regulations, and drivers didn't have to go through background checks or vehicle-safety inspections, which put consumers at risk.

We are still in the thick of understanding where artificial intelligence (AI) will take us, but we're already seeing a variety of serious concerns, including how bias can be baked into AI algorithms, which can affect everything from hiring decisions to policing to predicting patients' needs in the hospital.

Whenever a technology or innovation emerges that has the power to bring so much good into the world, things can go sideways in unexpected ways without the appropriate guardrails.

This is where we find the aesthetics industry today—and most patients are completely unaware of what's happening. Patients tend to assume that practitioners have a certain level of education, training, and proficiency. Getting 40 units of Botox from one clinic or med spa or another should be an apples-to-apples experience. And why would consumers think otherwise when this is how the medical industry has been set up to operate?

For example, if you were getting open-heart surgery, you would probably want to know how much training and experience your doctor had. But chances are you'd assume that if they're working as an open-heart surgeon, they must know what they're doing. You could take comfort in the fact that your doctor had to graduate from medical school, receive certain certifications, and continue adhering to strict standards for quality, both on a national level and through their hospital group. In other words, you wouldn't really have to vet your doctor because so many other individuals and groups were already putting in this work to make sure you're in good hands. The idea that someone could end up operating on you with zero formal education, little training, and no oversight from a governing body would be absurd.

Patients take this perspective into the realm of aesthetics. After all, many treatments are delivered in a healthcare setting by medical professionals.

But when it comes to aesthetics training and education, many patients would be shocked by how loosey-goosey the standards are for providing care. The person administering their injections might have very little experience with filler, despite being a licensed MD. Or they could get filler from a physician's assistant (PA) who has deep expertise and hundreds of hours of time on task—but isn't legally able to work in a neighboring state that doesn't allow PAs to provide that service.

As aesthetics professionals, we know how messy things have gotten behind the scenes. Everyone has an opinion on who should be allowed to provide what types of services and why. There's drama, controversy, and in-fighting.

First and foremost, the goal should be to take care of the patient. Instead of looking down our noses at each other, we should be reaching out with a helping hand to help rise up together.

How did we get here?

The aesthetics industry is a subset of the healthcare industry, but comparatively, it's just a baby. Cosmetic procedures used to live squarely in the realm of plastic surgery since treatments required cutting. But thanks to a variety of innovations with equipment, supplies, and techniques, we're now able to work a lot of magic without surgery.

As this happened, aesthetics expanded outside of plastics and into dermatology. This became a contentious situation for many years as plastic surgeons and dermatologists learned how to work alongside one another to help patients instead of seeing each other as competitors or adversaries. As more time passed, they came to realize that the demand for services was extensive—and they needed more hands at their practices. Plastic surgeons tend to prefer spending their time on treatments that use the full extent of their knowledge and training, so instead of taking the lead providing non-surgical treatments at their offices, they wanted to have their colleagues (those who were not MDs) take the lead and perform the services on their behalf. (And to be clear, this also happened in dermatology offices with derms wanting support from non-physician practitioners for less-invasive treatments.)

This is how businesses expand and grow in any industry; the founder alone cannot continue to take the lead providing every single service. Instead, they train and manage others who provide the services. This allows a business to increase its volume while also freeing up the founder's time for more complex and/or higher-revenue tasks, making the business more efficient and profitable.

But for this to work in aesthetics, non-physicians must have permission legally to practice. This is where issues around lobbying and licensing come into the picture. Lobbying efforts have often focused on state legislatures, where regulations about who can perform aesthetic procedures are determined. Physicians and their professional organizations began advocating for laws or regulations that allow nurses or PAs to perform specific treatments, such as injectables or laser treatments, under physician supervision or with minimal oversight.

There are a few different ways this has played out.

In some states, physicians can extend their licenses to non-physician practitioners, enabling them to perform aesthetic procedures in exchange for a fee or a percentage of the revenue. This arrangement benefits both parties economically: non-physicians gain access to a lucrative practice area while physicians earn passive income without directly performing the procedures.

In other states, lobbying efforts have led to the creation of collaborative practice agreements whereby physicians and nurses work together under a formal arrangement that allows nurses to perform a broader range of procedures. This type of agreement can streamline the process for nurses to offer treatments, especially in states with restrictive practice laws.

These lobbying efforts are often framed around ensuring patient safety while also increasing access to care. Proponents argue that allowing nurses and/or PAs to perform these procedures under the supervision of a physician ensures that patients receive safe, high-quality care while also expanding access to popular treatments.

The success of these lobbying efforts has varied by state, leading to a patchwork of regulations across the country. In some states, nurses and other non-physician practitioners have been granted broad authority to perform aesthetic procedures on their own or under the supervision of a physician, while in others, more restrictive rules remain in place.

Most everywhere these lobbying efforts have been successful, they have significantly impacted the dynamics and growth of the aesthetics industry.

While all this is going on, many physicians outside plastics and dermatology have also become interested in providing aesthetic services.

These professionals have undergone extensive training, including medical school, residency, and often fellowship training across various specialties. With a deep understanding of anatomy and medicine, branching into aesthetics, such as injectables, can seem like a relatively simple, natural, and profitable expansion. And of course, another factor at play here is the fact that non-physician practitioners were beginning to provide services in many states. Physicians thought, "Well, if they can do it, so can I."

With such a focus on what's happening in the United States, it can be easy for American practitioners to forget that there's a whole wide world outside the domestic aesthetics market. But the industry certainly is international, and millions of treatments around the globe are being led by professionals with a wide variety of educational backgrounds, certifications, and levels of experience.

I am in awe of some of these professionals! I follow them on social media, see them at conferences, and take part in the educational training sessions they offer. I've learned so much from many of these practitioners. It's interesting, though, because some of the world's aesthetics thought leaders and master injectors are not legally allowed to provide services in the United States, depending on their credentials and local laws. And yet many are asked to come to American conferences and trainings to share their knowledge and help train local practitioners—one more factor to muddy the waters on who should be allowed to provide what types of services and why.

Where does that leave us?

To be honest, it leaves us with a lot of confusion and conflicting opinions on who should be able to provide what types of services. This gray area has caused the atmosphere in the industry to become emotionally charged. Many of those who have more education and experience in aesthetics look down on those who are new to the field. And they don't even try to hide their disdain! Nurses and PAs know that many doctors not only do not respect them but also question whether they should be allowed to provide certain services. At the same time, physicians outside plastics and dermatology have gotten some side-eye from plastic surgeons and dermatologists for entering the space.

Let's be clear: looking down on anyone is disrespectful and wrong. None of us are perfect people, and riding a high horse doesn't help drive better outcomes for patients.

I'd like to challenge all practitioners in the industry to take a good look at confirmation bias. You can easily find plenty of examples that support your viewpoints, no matter what they are. If you believe that only someone with a certain license or educational background should be allowed to provide services, you can find horror stories that support your viewpoint. But it's essential to also be aware that there are plenty of examples that will contradict your viewpoint.

The reality is that the best aesthetic practitioners in the world are nothing if not diverse. Some are plastic surgeons; some are nurses. Some are MDs with deep education and experience across a range of specialties; some have chosen to hone in on a narrow specialty and develop niche expertise, such as lip injections. These professionals are incredibly different—and they should be valued for the excellent outcomes they can provide to patients. That's what we should be focusing on: outcomes.

Given the current state of the industry, how we can come together and support the best possible outcomes for patients?

Three things we can do

Standardize training requirements

We need to protect patients from unintended, yet foreseeable, impacts on safety and quality. We should all be able to agree that it's unsafe to provide aesthetic services without any training. Given this fact, we need to determine exactly how much training is appropriate for each type of service and ensure that all practitioners get this training before they work directly with patients. It sounds so simple, but doing so is a huge undertaking. The goal should be for everyone to have the same training regardless of their type of license, the state in which they practice, or how much experience they have.

At the same time, we also need training requirements to remain agile. With exponential advances in technology, training continues to be a moving target. The aesthetic services of today are not the same as 20, 10, or even 5 years ago. We aren't just cutting and using ablative lasers. Many, but not all, services still require broad and deep medical knowledge. For example, the newer lasers have advanced so much that they're essentially run by computer, so if a practitioner spends too much time in one area of skin, the machine will automatically turn off and thus avoid burning the patient. With this in mind, the time it takes to learn how to use one of these machines—and become good at it—is much less than in years past. As technology keeps advancing, training standards need to evolve as well so that it aligns with the times.

Be prepared to handle adverse outcomes

Dr. Jeanine Downie is a board-certified dermatologist who has been practicing medicine for decades, specializing in mostly cosmetic dermatology in her practice. Many of her patients have been with her for years, with her aesthetic patients coming in regularly for scheduled appointments.

She was surprised when a long-time patient of hers whom she hadn't seen in a while showed up at her office randomly with an acute care issue. The patient had gone to another doctor to get filler because their pricing was less expensive. Unfortunately, the doctor accidentally hit a blood vessel, and the patient was now experiencing a vascular occlusion (blocked blood vessel). She needed to be treated quickly or her tissue would die.

The patient said that the doctor who provided the filler wasn't able to help her. Dr. Downie was shocked. She promptly called the other doctor's office, an OB/GYN clinic, and asked why they were not able to treat the patient with Hylenex, an enzyme that dissolves hyaluronic-acid-based filler. Apparently, the doctor didn't keep Hylenex on site and never had training on how to administer it, as New Jersey does not require doctors to have treatments on hand to reverse the filler. (When practitioners purchase filler, they are required to sign a form that says they will always keep Hylenex on site, but many don't actually do it, and there's no governing body that performs site checks.)

Dr. Downie wanted to help the patient, but she understood that it could put her in a difficult position legally. She called her attorney, and he advised against offering any type of treatment. He said the patient could easily sue for what had already happened to her, and Dr. Downie would put herself at risk by getting involved. She felt terrible turning the patient away, especially since the patient needed Hylenex ASAP— and it takes two days or longer to have it shipped from a supplier, even if it's a rush order.

Dr. Downie ended up offering to sell the OB/GYN some of her Hylenex. This was a good workaround to offer to help without getting involved legally.

The patient went back to the other office and the doctor treated her, and, thankfully, she ended up being OK. (And, not surprisingly, the patient came back to Dr. Downie for all her aesthetic needs moving forward.)

This story shows how important it is for all practitioners to be prepared to handle adverse outcomes. It's not always possible for a patient to get help from someone else if things go wrong. Practitioners need to take that responsibility seriously.

I would love to see national regulation in this area. Practitioners should be faced with repercussions if they don't adhere to proper safety standards. But until this becomes law, the best we can do is hold ourselves and our colleagues to higher standards and educate our patients. Patients knowing what's at stake and feeling empowered to ask the right questions before getting services will only help push the industry in a safer direction.

Fight the black market

The black market for illegal knockoff drugs, including those of such popular medicines as Ozempic, Botox, and Juvéderm, is a growing concern, especially as demand for certain medications increases. These illegal markets often arise when a drug is expensive, difficult to obtain, or in high demand due to trends or off-label uses. These knockoff drugs

A New Frontier

As aesthetic practitioners, we find ourselves in a new frontier. With the lack of many formal regulations, we need to hold ourselves and our colleagues to high standards and have a solution-oriented mindset so that we can help move the industry in a safer direction.

may look similar to the genuine product but typically lack the authentic hologram, same active ingredients, proper dosage, and/or safety measures. In some cases, they may contain harmful substances or dangerous levels of key ingredients. According to a recent study, about 42 percent of online pharmacies that sell semaglutide (Ozempic) are illegal, operating without a valid license and selling medications without prescriptions.[11]

The global nature of the internet and the anonymity it offers make it challenging for regulatory bodies to police the sale of counterfeit drugs. These illegal operations are often sophisticated and able to evade detection by authorities. Though governments and regulatory agencies, such as the US Food and Drug Administration (FDA), are working to combat the spread of counterfeit drugs by tracking and shutting down illegal online pharmacies, increasing public awareness, and implementing stricter regulations on drug manufacturing and distribution, it remains all too easy for anyone with a credit card to purchase drugs on the black market. And many don't even understand that this is where the drugs are coming from!

Practitioners can lose their license if they purchase products from suppliers that are not licensed distributors. And if they're extending their license to nurses or PAs who then purchase products illegally, they could lose their license. I've seen it happen to people, and it's a terrible thing to go through. Even worse, what if one of those illegal medications kills someone and you're responsible? This is a very real outcome to consider.

It might be tempting to purchase drugs from unapproved sellers if you've heard from friends or colleagues that the products are real. But it's not worth the risk.

The government already has a number of processes in place to fight the black market, but a key strategy to help move things in a better direction is patient education. People need to be aware of the risks associated with purchasing medications from unverified sources and the importance of obtaining drugs through legitimate, regulated channels. Patients need to know that many practitioners buy from the black market (intentionally or unknowingly) to use at their clinics. This is a key reason not to choose your practitioner based on whoever has the lowest prices. Practitioners should proactively educate patients on where their drugs came from so they have the peace of mind that they are safe. Once this becomes normalized, the black market will lose its power.

CHAPTER 3

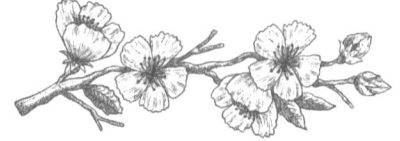

A New Approach

Many patients expect to walk into a clinic, get their Botox injections, and leave. They view the experience as a straightforward transaction rather than a comprehensive healthcare service. And this should come as no surprise since this is exactly what happens at many doctor's offices and med spas! But that's not how I run my practice. I believe in the power of holistic, highly personalized care because it's what's best for patients. In this chapter, I cover my approach and why it makes such a difference in outcomes.

The new-patient consultation

When it comes to most things in life, it's better to have a plan in place than needing to respond to issues as they come up. Unfortunately, in the world of aesthetics, it's common for patients to seek immediate, one-off solutions for specific concerns. But in so doing, they often fail to consider the broader context of their overall aesthetic goals or how specific treatments can fit into their journey.

That's why I always provide a full consultation to new patients before performing any services. This enables me to truly understand them and their needs and develop a personalized treatment plan. Though this may initially seem like extra work for practitioners or an unnecessary step to patients who are eager for quick treatments, it ensures that any service aligns with a patient's broader goals and delivers the best possible outcome.

A new-patient consultation adds an extra step for practitioners, and it also makes sense in terms of long-term planning and patient retention. We want to bring in new patients who stay with us rather than bounce around to different practices. By taking the time to get to know patients and show our expertise, we build a solid foundation for a relationship that will last.

Start by listening

Whenever a patient comes in for a consultation, I always ensure that they are the ones leading the conversation and sharing what concerns they have. I ask them to hold a mirror up to their face and tell me what bothers them. I do this because my job is not to critique patients or impose my own beauty standards or priorities onto them; rather, my job is to help patients feel better about themselves.

Practitioners should never tell patients that they can fix, change, or enhance something that the patient hasn't already brought up as an area of concern. Pointing out what we see as aesthetic deficiencies is hurtful. And when we stand to gain financially from patients being troubled by additional aspects of their appearance, driving the conversation on what areas to focus on is manipulative and unethical.

Most practitioners do not have this malicious intent. However, it's easy to hastily make comments to patients that can have major consequences in how they see themselves. It is important that these practitioners keep in mind that the patients who are coming to see them already critique themselves in the mirror every day. There is something about their appearance that is bothering them deeply enough that they are willing to spend hard-earned money and time and go through physical pain to improve their emotional state. The last thing they need is to be told that they should be worried about additional aspects of their appearance.

Sometimes it can be difficult to bite your tongue during consultations when patients do not bring up the areas of concern that you anticipate, but you must. You might think you're doing patients a favor by letting them know other ways you could change their appearance, but it's crucial to realize that your perspective is unique to you. You live in a beauty bubble based on your upbringing, culture, and social circle. But there isn't one right answer when it comes to beauty. Some people want full lips and others couldn't care less. Some want nothing more than to be a size 2, and others strive for as much volume as possible in their derriere. More power to all these people! Our job isn't to push them in a certain direction when it comes to how they look. Our job is to help them get to where *they* want to go.

Be the expert

Let's pretend that one day you're driving home from work and your car starts making a deafening clanking sound. You pull into a mechanic's shop to get some help and, like most people, probably expect the mechanic to take a look at the car and advise you on how they would fix the issue. But what if they didn't? What if they simply asked you what part you wanted them to replace? You'd probably wonder how in the world they stay in business, and then you'd go somewhere else.

Whether it's an auto mechanic, a plumber, or a surgeon, you expect service-practitioner experts to use their knowledge to advise you on how to move forward. The same should be true in the world of aesthetics. Patients might come in with an idea for how to get the results they want, but they are not the expert.

I'll be honest: there are a lot of nuances when it comes to stepping into the role of the expert. There's a balance between listening to what patients say they want and understanding the best possible pathways to achieve those results. Often, patients come into my office and say that they want a specific treatment. But their understanding of aesthetic dermatology is limited, and what they are asking for might not be the best option for achieving their desired results. Instead of simply providing the thing they ask for, it's my job to ask questions to understand their needs and guide them in the best possible direction to reach their goals. Sometimes this

There's a balance between listening to what patients say they want and understanding the best possible pathways to achieve those results.

means recommending a totally different treatment modality or plan. Maybe they are ready to buy microneedling but a laser treatment is a better fit. Practitioners cannot shy away from making this type of recommendation.

Other times, giving an honest recommendation means turning people away. For example, I sometimes refer patients to a plastic surgeon who can better meet their needs. I typically do this when it would be difficult to achieve the patient's desired results through the treatment options I provide. For example, if someone wants more-youthful-looking skin and it would require routine laser treatments or many vials of filler, it could make more sense to opt for a facelift instead. I present this option to patients so they can make an informed decision. Some people see a facelift as a simpler solution than coming in repeatedly to make incremental progress over time. Other people have an aversion to any type of cutting or going under anesthesia and prefer to avoid plastic surgery at all costs.

Sometimes patients are interested in results that simply aren't realistic through aesthetic treatments or plastic surgery. This mostly happens with older patients. But because I don't want them to waste their time and money and go through any discomfort only to be unsatisfied with the results, I'm always very up-front with them about what they can expect.

I recently had a woman who was in her 70s come in to see me, and she asked me what I could do about her wrinkles. Her skin quality was good for her age, and in reality, she was just at that point in her life when human beings have wrinkles. I told her that I thought she was beautiful and wouldn't recommend any services. She thanked me and said that was all she needed to hear.

Getting the consultation right is a key part of the job that differentiates the masters from the technicians.

Conduct an initial assessment

In aesthetics, it's important to start with a clear understanding of your patient's skin. This can be done through good old-fashioned observation, but technology can truly take this to the next level.

The Visia machine is an advanced imaging system that I swear by for performing comprehensive full-face assessments. It provides a detailed analysis of the skin's condition by capturing high-resolution images of the face and using specialized software to evaluate various aspects of skin health. This ensures that the consultation is rooted in science rather than subjective opinion. Here's how it works:

- Multi-spectral imaging: The Visia machine captures images of the face using different types of light, including standard, cross-polarized, and UV. These different lighting conditions allow the machine to visualize and assess various skin features that are not always visible to the naked eye.
- 3-D imaging: Certain models of the Visia system can create 3-D images of the face, providing a more detailed view of facial contours and structure. This can be especially useful for assessing the results of volume-related treatments or planning procedures that affect facial symmetry.

These images provide a comprehensive skin analysis:

- Wrinkles and fine lines: The Visia system can detect and quantify the depth and extent of wrinkles and fine lines, providing a clear picture of aging signs.
- Texture and pores: The machine assesses skin texture and pore size, helping to identify areas of roughness and/or enlarged pores that might benefit from treatments.
- Pigmentation and sun damage: The system can highlight areas of hyperpigmentation, sun damage, and UV spots that are not visible under normal light. This helps practitioners understand the extent of sun damage.
- Redness and vascular conditions: The machine also identifies areas of redness or visible blood vessels, which can be important for diagnosing conditions such as rosacea or planning treatments.

After the assessment, the Visia system generates detailed reports that summarize the findings. One of the most interesting and valuable benefits of the machine is the comparative analysis it provides. The

Visia system includes a database that allows practitioners to compare a patient's skin condition with others in their age group or skin type. This comparative analysis can help show how their skin health ranks relative to their peers, making an objective case for recommended treatments. (Going by a patient's age alone doesn't always work well for assessments because skin quality can be so different. Knowing the "Visia age" has been valuable for me when it comes to predicting how patients will respond to various treatments.)

The machine's visual outputs are powerful tools for patient education. Seeing detailed images and data about their skin can help patients understand the need for certain treatments, making them more likely to commit to a comprehensive skincare plan recommended by their practitioner.

The Visia machine cost my practice about $20,000, which certainly isn't peanuts, but it has been well worth the investment. It is impossible for me to see the extent of skin damage with the naked eye, and the machine helps me see what's really happening on and under the top layer of the dermis. I've found that this comprehensive assessment has enabled me to develop more-personalized treatment plans and track the effectiveness of interventions, leading to more-informed decisions and better patient outcomes.

The machine can also be used in follow-up visits to track the progress of treatments. By comparing before and after images and data, practitioners are able to objectively show the effectiveness of the treatments, which helps in patient satisfaction and ongoing care planning.

If you don't have a Visia machine, you should still onboard new patients with a full-face consultation and develop an aesthetics plan for the year. Even if your patients have not asked for and therefore are not expecting it, it's what they want.

After the initial consultation and plan, make sure you stay in the driver's seat for guiding your patients. One of my friends told me how she has been going to her gynecologist for Botox for the past couple years. Each visit starts with her gynecologist asking her if she wants the same thing as last time. My friend has said yes to this maybe six or seven times, and now she's starting to wonder if she should be asking for something else and what that might be. But of course, she doesn't know what she doesn't know!

All too often, practitioners of any service look to the customer to guide the process despite the customer lacking the knowledge to fully understand what they need or want. Don't fall into this trap. Of course, patients' wishes must always be respected, but that does not make them the expert in the relationship—even if they've been coming to you for years. They are seeking the best possible outcomes, and that will not be achieved if they are put in the position of guiding the aesthetic treatment process. It's time for all practitioners to step into the role of being the expert, rather than just a technician who is executing the service requested by the patient.

Focus on holistic care

The body is a complex system. Everything is connected. Unfortunately, Western medicine isn't set up to focus on holistic health. Instead, it's siloed off into specialties and sub-specialties that often don't collaborate well. On top of that, Western medicine is also reactive. Patients come in with problems and doctors are tasked with fixing them. In this system, there is no incentive to keep patients well. As a result, Americans have shockingly poor health when you consider how much money goes into healthcare.

This might sound lofty, but I truly believe that aesthetic practitioners can help guide healthcare in a better direction and move the needle on wellness. Hear me out.

One of the best ways to keep patients healthy is by increasing the number of touch points they have with wellness experts. (Note that I didn't specifically say "doctors" here. I said "wellness experts.") What exactly is a wellness expert? We could argue it in many different directions, but for our purposes here, it means anyone who has knowledge that can help patients improve their health. In some cases, this might mean noticing malignant melanoma skin cancer. In other cases, it might mean seeing that the patient looks tired and talking with them about the importance of getting more sleep.

Sometimes the advice, tips, or suggestions people need to hear isn't the kind of information that's going to change the world. Sometimes it can easily be found by Googling or asking Alexa. Many times, it's common sense. But that doesn't mean it isn't valuable.

Studies show that people often need to hear a message numerous times before it sinks in and they decide to alter their behavior. With this in mind, aesthetic practitioners are well positioned to offer holistic wellness support through additional touch points along a patient's regular care journey. While patients might see their general practitioner once a year, they could see an aesthetic practitioner much more frequently.

On top of this, small changes can make a huge impact over time. Getting people thinking about the little things they can do to look and feel their best creates a ripple effect that changes everything.

I've seen this firsthand at my clinic. As a dermatologist, I provide both medical and aesthetic services; some of my patients are purely medical, some are purely aesthetic, and some cross over into both realms. I've noticed that most of my aesthetic patients practice self-care much better than most of my patients who only come in for purely medical services do. When I ask my aesthetic patients about their wellness habits, they often tell me that they eat healthy, exercise regularly, get good sleep, and even meditate. My medical patients tend to be less proactive about self-care, and it shows in their skin, as well as their health overall.

All this sounds so logical, right?

More effort -> better outcomes

This is why all practitioners should all be asking how they can do a little more to help their aesthetic patients when they walk through the door. It's not just about executing a one-off service or thinking about the skin as an isolated area of health. They need to look at patients holistically and do their best to help them, wherever they are. There are many things that people can do easily, for free, that make a noticeable difference in how they look and feel.

For example, drinking enough water truly does not get the credit it deserves. We all know that water is healthy and we should probably drink more of it, but most patients aren't aware that it really makes a difference in how youthful their skin looks on any given day. I can tell if someone is well hydrated just by looking at them. Other major factors that are often overlooked in the beauty world are stress and sleep. People who go through a lot of stress tend to get more wrinkles earlier. Lack of sleep creates bags under the eyes and can make the skin dull.

We are doing patients an incredible disservice if we ignore these kinds of factors when they come in for our help. It's our job to make sure patients know that the skin is a window into overall wellness. When the skin isn't looking its best, there are likely many things that could help.

The next few chapters are dedicated to the simple things that people can do to take care of their skin envelope outside of aesthetic treatments. I recommend sharing as much of this information as you can with patients during the initial consultation, as well as reminding patients of the best practices whenever they come in for treatments. If we consider ourselves to be aesthetic artists, when our patients take better care of themselves, we have a higher-quality canvas to work with. And more importantly, addressing the issues that affect the skin makes a huge impact in our patients' health overall.

CHAPTER 4

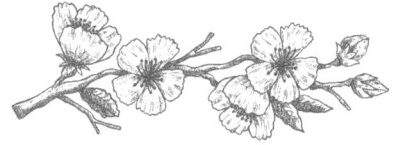

Vitamins and Nutrition

Before we get into all the amazing aesthetic dermatology treatments that are available today, we need to start with the basics. Fueling the body with the proper vitamins and nutrients can make a major difference in both physical health and appearance.

It baffles me how little this is talked about in dermatology! I see patients all the time who would feel better and be more positive about how they look if they became intentional about nutrition. This is true for people who have certain skin conditions (e.g., psoriasis, eczema, acne) as well as those who don't. Vitamins and proper nutrition should be considered the low-hanging fruit for dermatology. It's not overly expensive, invasive, or difficult to start here. And it's a solid investment in your personal health and well-being. In this chapter, I go over what you need to know about taking care of yourself from the inside out.

Following guidelines and research

Whenever we're making decisions about our health, it's important to use research and follow guidelines from experts. As a science nerd, I love reading research papers and studies to learn about new findings. Science is an ever-evolving field. As an international community, we learn new things every single day. For this reason, guidelines and recommendations are never static. Instead, they are often a moving target based on what new research uncovers. But it's important to note that guidelines can't be updated immediately based on a single study, or even many studies. Governing bodies are conservative, and they safeguard against giving people incorrect advice. Unfortunately, this often causes a different problem. When new evidence strongly points toward updating guidelines, it can take years for these agencies to get on board, fully support the research, and update their recommendations.

Another interesting factor here is that when the government updates certain guidelines for health, it must also update many other laws and processes to match so that it isn't publicly saying one thing but doing another. For example, if new research showed that kids shouldn't be eating more than 20 grams of sugar per day but the public-school lunches being served across the nation (and funded by the government) exceeded that amount, there could be a problem. Since it would take time and money for school lunches to catch up to the new, healthier guidelines, the government would be motivated to move slower in terms of making those changes. It's unfortunate, but this happens all the time, in many ways.

Additionally, if you compare guidelines from various governing bodies and agencies in the United States and abroad, you'll notice that recommendations aren't exactly the same. That's why it's important to understand the guidelines, discuss concerns with your healthcare practitioner, and stay informed on recent research that is likely to disrupt any advice you've been following. From there, you can make your own decisions on what makes the most sense, given lifestyle factors and risk tolerance.

As an aesthetic practitioner, it's especially important for you to level up your knowledge on nutraceuticals so you can best advise your patients. There will be many opportunities for you to provide recommendations and suggestions that could be just as powerful as the aesthetic treatments you provide.

How to take vitamins

Know how much your body needs. Check the guidelines from various governing bodies on the recommended number of milligrams for vitamins and supplements based on your gender and age. This is a good place to start when it comes to determining what your body needs. Note that your existing health conditions, current prescriptions, and other factors affect these recommendations.

If you're experiencing a specific health issue that concerns you, it might make sense to get a blood test that assesses your levels of various vitamins so that you can determine whether you have a deficiency. For example, I order tests when people are experiencing hair loss. Based on the results, I can often tell that increasing levels of certain vitamins can help support better outcomes.

Before you begin taking any new supplements, make sure you talk with your healthcare practitioner about what makes sense for you given your unique medical history and needs. Lastly, be aware that many nutraceuticals can have adverse effects if they are consumed in large quantities or if they're mixed with certain medications.[12]

Determine if you can get your recommended vitamins from food. The best way to get your vitamins is directly through food rather than supplements. Whole foods contain a variety of vitamins, minerals, fiber, and other bioactive compounds that work together synergistically. This synergy can enhance the absorption and effectiveness of nutrients. A diet rich in colorful fruits, vegetables (especially leafy greens), whole grains, lean proteins, beans, lentils, and healthy fats provides a wide array of nutrients that support overall health.

If you're having trouble getting enough vitamins from your diet, try cutting back on the foods that don't have much nutritional value in order to make room for healthier choices.

Understand cofactors. Cofactors are substances that assist in the biochemical reactions of vitamins within the body. Vitamins often need cofactors in order to work properly and help enzymes (special proteins) carry out such essential tasks as making energy, repairing cells, and keeping our metabolism running smoothly. Without enough vitamins and their cofactors, our bodies can't function properly, leading to problems such as low energy, a weak immune system, and slow healing. In addition to getting the milligrams you need for the vitamins you're targeting, you want to make sure you have the proper cofactors so that your body can get maximum benefit from the vitamins.

Make a plan for getting the remaining amount from supplements. Taking vitamins seems straightforward, but it's not. That's because vitamins are absorbed differently into the body depending on what they interact with in your stomach, fatty tissue, and liver. You can take a vitamin every single day at the wrong time and get zero benefit from it. And many people do just that. What a waste!

Some doctors recommend taking a multivitamin. Based on research, the jury is still out on whether doing so makes a difference in various health outcomes. When it comes to skincare, which is my overall focus in this book, there are specific vitamins I recommend. But if you had to choose between eating a colorful plate of food and the individual nutraceuticals featured in this chapter, know that you are likely to get better results by focusing on your diet. Put your efforts there! Nutraceuticals are supplemental.

For each of my recommendations, I've included the most important things you need to know about how and when to take the nutraceuticals so that your body can fully absorb them.

Buy high-quality products. The supplement industry hasn't been as regulated as it should be, and not all products are created equal. Without strict regulations, there is variability in the purity and potency of vitamins and minerals found in supplements. Some products may contain lower amounts of active ingredients than stated on the label, or they may include impurities and contaminants. Additionally, the form of vitamins used in supplements can affect their absorption and effectiveness in the body. Some forms of vitamins may not be verified or as bioavailable, meaning that the body cannot absorb and utilize them as effectively as it can higher-quality forms. The Mayo Clinic recommends looking for independent assessments of quality, such as the United States Pharmacopeia (USP) symbol, which indicates that a supplement meets USP standards for strength and purity. Other seals that verify a product's ingredients and safety include NSF, UL (formerly known as Underwriters Laboratories), and ConsumerLab.com.[13,14]

Don't rely on topical vitamins. You will often see vitamins sold in various formats such as lotions or balms that promise that they can be absorbed through the skin. Many times, this is false advertising as it's actually quite complicated for topical products to get through the skin—and for good reason! There are many layers that protect your body from the outside world. That's why it's often better to take your vitamins through food, science-based medical-grade skincare treatments, and oral supplements.

Note that certain topical products do contain vitamins that are absorbed into the skin, such as vitamin C serums, but they are not a substitute for getting vitamin C from your diet. More on this in chapter 6.

Recommended vitamins for skin

Vitamin D

This is the number-one vitamin I recommend to my patients, for a variety of reasons. Vitamin D plays a key role in skin-cell growth and repair, which is exactly what helps your face look years younger. Before you invest money in more expensive aesthetic treatments, take your vitamins! As a board-certified dermatologist, I recognize and understand that our academy follows the National Academy of Medicine, formerly the Institute of Medicine. The Academy's stance—at least at the time of this writing—is that vitamin D has only been proven to be beneficial for bone health. That said, research continues, and I am interested in continuing the conversation shaped by newer studies and look forward to updated guidelines. As far as vitamin D goes, chances are that you need it. The World Health Organization has determined that a good portion of the population has insufficient levels of vitamin D.[15] (And this is considering the current guidelines, which have not been updated since 2011 and are likely considerably lower than they should be given recent research.[16,17,18,19]) This is a troubling fact as newer studies link low levels of vitamin D to an increased risk of serious conditions and diseases such as Alzheimer's, Parkinson's, cancer (at least 15 types), type 2 diabetes, depression, schizophrenia, poor bone health, heart disease, autoimmune diseases, and hair loss—just to name a few.[20,21,22]

If you are already suffering from some of these conditions, there's a chance that vitamin D could help you feel better. For example, I've seen psoriasis go away after patients increased their levels of vitamin D. There might not be conclusive evidence (yet) on how vitamin D can help with various health conditions, but it's smart to go out of your way to make sure your levels aren't low.

You might be wondering whether you can get enough of your vitamin D from the sun. Studies have shown that anywhere from 5 to 30 minutes (depending on skin type and the latitude where you live) of sunshine per day is enough to activate your body's production of vitamin D, but the interesting thing is that sun exposure beyond this timeframe has been proven to actually deplete your level of vitamin D.[23]

- How to take vitamin D: It's fat soluble, which means you should always take it with food or right after eating. I recommend not combining it with calcium when taking high-level vitamin D supplementation. Vitamin D toxicity can occur with high levels of calcium in the blood, and taking the vitamin as a supplement can lead to potential kidney problems, including kidney stones.[24] Certain medications such as antacids and Lipitor can prevent healthy absorption. Cofactors including vitamin K, zinc, boron, and vitamin A can help absorb vitamin D.
- Foods rich in vitamin D: These include fatty fish (e.g., salmon and mackerel), cod liver oil, canned tuna, egg yolks, fortified dairy products, fortified plant-based milk, fortified orange juice, fortified breakfast cereals, and mushrooms.

Vitamin B3

Consuming adequate amounts of vitamin B3 (niacinamide, or niacin) through your diet can positively impact your skin health. Niacin enhances your skin barrier by promoting ceramide production, helping retain moisture and protect against environmental damage. Its anti-inflammatory properties help manage skin conditions such as acne, eczema, and psoriasis, while its effect on improved blood circulation delivers oxygen and nutrients to the skin, promoting a healthy complexion. Niacin supports collagen and elastin synthesis, reducing the appearance of fine lines and wrinkles. It also aids in DNA repair, protecting against UV damage and reducing the risk of sunburn and photoaging. Niacin also regulates sebaceous-gland activity, preventing excess oil production and breakouts.

A study in the *New England Journal of Medicine* shows that taking 500 mg twice a day is associated with a 23-percent decrease in pre-cancers.[25]

- How to take vitamin B3: B vitamins are water soluble, which means the body does not store them. You can take them with or without food. B vitamins are said to provide energy, so it's often recommended to take them in the morning. It is rare for anyone in the developed world to have a B3 deficiency, although in the United States, alcoholism is a main cause of it.[26] Cofactors for B3 include tryptophan, vitamin B2, vitamin B6, iron, magnesium, and zinc.

- Foods rich in B3: These include beets, chicken, turkey, tuna, salmon, beef, pork, brown rice, peanuts, avocado, and mushrooms.

Zinc

Zinc is an essential mineral that significantly benefits skin health. It accelerates wound healing by aiding collagen synthesis and cell proliferation, making it crucial for repairing cuts and abrasions. Its anti-inflammatory properties and ability to reduce sebum production help treat acne and inflammatory skin conditions such as eczema and rosacea. As an antioxidant, zinc protects skin cells from free radicals and UV damage, reducing premature aging and skin-cancer risk. It regulates sebaceous glands, preventing excess oil and clogged pores, and supports collagen and elastin production, thereby helping to maintain skin firmness and elasticity. Zinc also helps dark spots fade by inhibiting excess melanin production. Lastly, and perhaps most interestingly, zinc helps Botox last longer.[27]

- How to take zinc: Your body absorbs 20 to 40 percent of the zinc present in food. So even if you think you're eating plenty of zinc, you're not benefiting from anywhere near the full amount. Zinc from animal proteins is more readily absorbed by the body than is zinc from plant foods. To increase your absorption from zinc supplements, take them with meals that contain protein. Cofactors include vitamin A, vitamin B6, and magnesium.

- Foods rich in zinc: These include oysters, beef, crab, lobster, pork, chicken, pumpkin seeds, chickpeas, cashews, yogurt, and cheese.

Omega-3s

Omega-3 fatty acids are essential for maintaining healthy skin. They strengthen the skin's barrier function, helping to retain moisture and protect against irritants and pollutants. Their anti-inflammatory properties reduce redness and irritation, which are beneficial for conditions such as acne, eczema, and psoriasis. Omega-3s also support the production of collagen, enhancing skin elasticity and reducing the appearance of fine lines and wrinkles. They improve blood flow, delivering essential nutrients and oxygen to the skin, promoting a healthy, radiant complexion. Omega-3s protect against UV-induced damage from sun exposure, reducing the risk of sunburn and photoaging. Furthermore, in a recently published study, patients with moderate to severe acne who were given high levels of omega-3 demonstrated a decrease in their clinical appearance of acne.[28]

- How to take omega-3s: Omega-3s are fat soluble and better absorbed when taken with dietary fats. Cofactors include vitamin E, vitamin C, B vitamins, magnesium, and zinc.
- Foods rich in omega-3s: These include fatty fish (e.g., salmon and mackerel), flaxseeds, chia seeds, walnuts, hemp seeds, anchovies, brussels sprouts, seaweed, and edamame.

Vitamin K

Vitamin K is essential for maintaining healthy skin by aiding in the body's natural blood-clotting process, which helps heal wounds and reduce bruising. It supports the skin's ability to repair itself and minimizes the appearance of scars and dark circles under the eyes. Additionally, vitamin K helps improve skin elasticity and may reduce the appearance of fine lines and wrinkles. Its anti-inflammatory properties can also help reduce redness and irritation.

- How to take vitamin K: It's fat soluble so it's better absorbed when taken with dietary fats. If you're on blood-thinning medication, it can potentially interfere, so be sure to consult a doctor.
- Foods rich in vitamin K: These include leafy green vegetables, cruciferous vegetables, parsley, cilantro, eggs, kiwi, and avocado.

Collagen and amino acids

Collagen is a vital protein that forms the structural framework of the skin, helping to maintain its firmness and smoothness. As we age, collagen production naturally decreases, leading to wrinkles, sagging, and dryness. By consuming collagen-rich foods and/or supplements, you can support your skin's structure, elasticity, and hydration. Additionally, collagen-rich diets may support the body's natural defenses against oxidative stress and inflammation, which contribute to premature aging and skin damage.

Some people swear by taking collagen supplements, and a recent meta-analysis of 26 studies shows some benefit of hydrolyzed collagen (HC) versus a placebo. However, there were no significant differences between the sources of HC, and a review of these studies further shows that biases in the current studies exist as well. Given the lack of conclusive evidence on how effective collagen supplements are for the skin, it appears that the body's ability to absorb collagen through pills and powders isn't as high as many collagen-supplement companies want people to believe.[29] This is especially important to note because out of all the supplements I recommend in this chapter, collagen supplements are the most expensive.

Luckily, there are great options for getting what you need through your diet. Collagen is made up of amino acids, so focusing on eating plenty of amino acids can have the same effect on your skin as consuming collagen directly.

- Foods rich in collagen: These include fish skin and bone broth from beef, chicken, or pork.
- Foods rich in amino acids: These include chicken, turkey, quinoa, tofu, eggs, salmon, tuna, Greek yogurt, lentils, almonds, and chia seeds.

Polypodium leucotomos

This product can be a godsend for people with fair skin! Heliocare is the brand name of this over-the-counter dietary supplement that provides an added layer of protection from the sun. It contains an extract from the fern *Polypodium leucotomos*, which comes from Central and South America. Research shows that it offers a range of benefits, including acting as a scavenger in the body to mop up free radicals, thereby reducing oxidative stress and skin aging. It also protects against the harmful effects of UV radiation, thereby safeguarding against sunburns.[30]

- How to take Heliocare: Heliocare should be used in conjunction with topical sunscreens. It is not a replacement. Heliocare is safe to take every day, or you can simply take it before you know you're going to spend time in the sun. This helps protect against sunburn for about two hours. (Antioxidant properties continue working beyond this time frame.)

Personalize your diet

In addition to getting your vitamins, your overall diet has an impact on your skin. Eating healthy makes a difference, but there's no "one-size-fits-all" approach to nutrition. Not everyone is meant to eat every food. Based on genetics and other individual factors, we don't all have the same enzymes. That means there are real biological differences in how people digest various foods and absorb nutrients. Foods that are perfect fuel for one person can make another person feel terrible.

It's important to understand what works for your body. Not only is this crucial for your health overall, but it makes a difference for your skin. When you can't digest certain things, it affects the texture, coloring, moisture level, and general health of your skin. For example, some people who suffer from rough, scaly skin have an underlying issue with their ability to process vitamin A. Those who suffer from acne experience breakouts that are linked to eating dairy. In either of these situations, treating the skin alone is not an effective way to solve the problem in the long term. That's why it's worth the time and effort to assess your diet and ensure that food isn't the root cause of any troubling health symptoms.

I was having some health issues a few years ago that I suspected were linked to food and supplements I was taking, so I decided to go to the Mayo Clinic for help. My doctor gave me incredible advice. He said that if something doesn't make me feel good when I eat it, I shouldn't be eating it. If I feel bloated or mentally foggy after a meal, it's a bad sign. He recommended a food diary and cutting out those triggering foods from my diet, reintroducing them one at a time, seeing how I feel, and then deciding from there whether to keep those foods in my diet. I followed his advice, and that's how I realized that I feel much better when I don't eat a lot of gluten and cut out unregulated supplements.

It's important to realize that what we choose to eat in our day-to-day lives is highly personal. Summer is the most beautiful time of year in the Black Hills where we live, and we tend to host a lot of family and friends here during that time of year. At our home, we try to eat seasonal whole foods, which is based on the good advice I was given by an acupuncturist friend over a decade ago. When my friends and family were last visiting, I noticed in the quiet, beautiful morning hours here that almost everyone in our circle started their day with a caffeinated coffee. For me, it's a double espresso—however, sometimes it's more—and most of our guests would gather around our coffee maker and chat to start the day.

Lucky for us, a recent study found that those drinking four of more cups of coffee per day were significantly less likely to report having been diagnosed with rosacea.[31] What I think is most interesting about this is that it might underscore the importance of eating and drinking that which makes you feel good. My Northern European DNA is highly prone to rosacea, and maybe my ritual of caffeinated coffee over the years has been protective.

Another example of food having protective properties, and something I have always gravitated toward as my preferred sweetener, is honey. A study on bee products in dermatology highlights their biological properties—related to the flavonoids they contain—that are used to heal burns and are antibiotic, anti-inflammatory, antioxidant, antifungal, antiviral, and more.[32]

> *By prioritizing internal nutrition before focusing on aesthetic treatments, people can achieve more sustainable and effective results as the skin's underlying health is improved, making it more receptive to external treatments.*

Speaking of sweets, there's one thing I advise all my patients to cut back on in order to protect their skin: sugar. A study featured in the *Journal of Drugs and Dermatology* shows that when sugar is metabolized into your cells, particularly your skin, it causes loss of elasticity (e.g., aging). In fact, it can accumulate in your cells and make them older than other cells.[33] And remember that carbs are essentially sugars, so as much as we don't want to hear it, cutting way back on sugar/carbs is smart for the skin.

What are your favorite foods? Have you spent any time reflecting on how they make you feel and whether they are benefitting you and your special needs?

It's time to take a holistic approach to skin health—especially in the realm of aesthetics. Healthy skin starts from the inside out. By prioritizing internal nutrition before focusing on aesthetic treatments, people can achieve more sustainable and effective results as the skin's underlying health is improved, making it more receptive to external treatments.

If you are an aesthetic practitioner, it's your responsibility to make sure your patients understand the power of vitamins and nutrition.

It takes knowledge, intentionality, and dedication to continuously implement all the advice in this chapter, but I can promise you that it's worth it. Every little bit counts. Don't get discouraged if you fall behind on your vitamins or fall off the wagon with your diet. Give yourself grace and get back to it!

CHAPTER 5

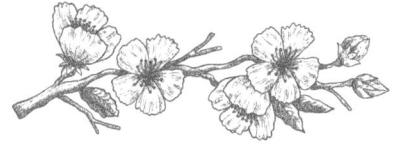

Sun Protection

The easiest thing you can do to keep your skin healthy and beautiful is to protect it from the sun. I cannot drive this point home hard enough! Shade is your friend! My nonprofit organization, Made for Shade, was founded on this simple principle. It feels good to spend time in the sun, and I'm not saying that people should completely avoid it. But there's an enormous amount of evidence that shows a clear cause-and-effect relationship between sun exposure and skin health. More than 90 percent of skin cancers are caused by sun exposure.[34] One out of five Americans will develop skin cancer by age 70.[35]

In addition to causing serious health concerns, nothing ages the skin faster than the sun. A year of poor sun protection on the face can make someone look a decade older. Of course, there are treatments to help revitalize the skin and bring back a more youthful appearance, and we'll get to that later in this book, but turning back the hands of time isn't necessarily easy. It's always smarter to hold onto what you have for as long as you can in order to reduce your need for treatment.

The value of sun protection has become widely accepted today, but there's a major lack of understanding of how people can protect themselves. Some of this confusion stems from how skincare treatments and recommendations have evolved over the past couple decades due to new research. Combine this with misleading marketing messaging around sunscreen, not to mention influencers spreading misinformation on social media, and people don't know what to believe anymore. Most individuals care about their health enough to make good choices, but the limiting factor in taking the right actions is education.

The knowledge you will gain from this chapter will help you make improvements that will not only keep you looking years younger but also potentially add years to your life. No matter how easily you burn or how old you are, sun protection is your cornerstone for aesthetics. There's no point even talking about advanced aesthetic dermatology treatments if you haven't already covered your bases with sun protection.

If you're an aesthetic practitioner, you have a responsibility to make sure your patients are well informed on how to protect themselves. Don't assume that they already know what to do. Most don't. They're looking to you for advice on how to improve their skin—and proper sun protection is the foundation.

Understanding rays

Ultraviolet

The rays that are most well known are ultraviolet (UV) rays. They are primarily divided into two types: UVA and UVB. Both types of rays damage the skin, albeit in different ways.

UVA: UVA rays penetrate deeply into the skin, leading to premature aging by breaking down collagen and elastin, which results in wrinkles and sagging skin. Unlike UVB, which causes direct DNA damage, UVA rays induce DNA damage indirectly by creating reactive oxygen species. This indirect damage can cause mutations over time, increasing the risk of skin cancer, including melanoma. UVA exposure can lead to hyperpigmentation and the formation of dark spots and age spots, as it stimulates the production of melanin.

UVA rays are present during all daylight hours and can even penetrate clouds and glass. This means your skin is exposed to UVA rays even on cloudy days or when indoors near windows.

The damaging effects of UVA rays weren't discovered until the 1990s. Before then, tanning-bed and -booth manufacturers had figured out how to remove the UVB rays so people could get a base tan easier without getting burned, yet they soon found out that users were getting cancer at disturbingly high rates.[36]

UVB: These rays penetrate through the outer layers of the skin and are the primary source of sunburns. UVB rays can directly damage the DNA in skin cells, increasing the risk of skin cancer, including melanoma, basal-cell carcinoma, and squamous-cell carcinoma.

UVB intensity varies according to the time of day, season, and your geographical location. It is strongest between 10 a.m. and 2 p.m. each day, during the summer months, and closer to the equator.

UV exposure increases when you're near reflective surfaces such as water, sand, or snow. Daily variations in the UV index, a measurement of the level of UV radiation that reaches the Earth's surface, make a difference as well, so it's a good idea to pay attention to that and avoid the sun whenever it reads as "high."

Infrared radiation

A lot of people are unfamiliar with infrared radiation (IR). These rays penetrate deeper than UV rays, reaching the dermis layer of the skin. IR is the reason your skin feels warm in the sun. Unlike with UVA and UVB rays, you experience IR from human-made sources such as heated metals, molten glass, home electrical appliances, incandescent bulbs, radiant heaters, furnaces, welding arcs, and plasma torches.[37] IR generates free radicals, leading to oxidative stress, inflammation, and the breakdown of collagen, all of which contribute to aging.

Visible light

High-energy visible (HEV) light, also known as blue light, is emitted by both the sun and electronic devices such as smartphones and computers. Although you won't get a burn from HEV light, it can penetrate the skin more deeply than UV rays can, causing oxidative stress and inflammation and potentially contributing to hyperpigmentation and aging.

Sunscreen

Sun-protection factor

Commonly known as SPF, the sun-protection factor is the number-one thing most people look for when they choose a sunscreen. SPF matters, but a lot of people don't realize that it's only part of the full sun-protection picture. The number associated with SPF is a measure of how well a sunscreen can protect the skin from UVB radiation. SPF does nothing against UVA rays, IR, or HEV.

The protection levels for SPF are a ratio that compares the amount of UV radiation required to cause sunburn on protected skin versus unprotected skin. For example, SPF 30 means that it takes 30 times longer for the skin to burn with sunscreen than without it.

Protection levels

SPF 15: Blocks approximately 93% of UVB rays (this is not enough protection for anyone on a long-term basis)
SPF 30: Blocks about 97% of UVB rays
SPF 50: Blocks about 98% of UVB rays
SPF 100: Blocks about 99% of UVB rays (higher SPF numbers offer slightly more protection, but none offer 100% protection)

Broad-spectrum sunscreen

Broad-spectrum sunscreen protects against both UVA and UVB rays. It does not protect against IR or HEV light. In the United States, if a bottle of sunscreen does not specifically say it's broad spectrum, there's no reason to assume it is.

To make things even more confusing, not all broad-spectrum sunscreens offer the same protection for UVA rays—even when comparing products with the same SPF. One brand might have 30 SPF and 30 UVA protection, and another might have 30 SPF and 5 UVA protection. This is an area where lack of regulation is literally killing people!

In the European Union and Australia, sunscreen regulations and standards are more stringent, which helps ensure that consumers are adequately protected from both types of harmful UV radiation. Here in the States, approvals from the FDA are slow, but our standards for testing sunscreens are often higher and stricter. This can be frustrating for those in our industry bringing new innovations to our consumers. Yet that is our current reality—and it's good that you're doing your own research.

Mineral sunscreens vs. chemical sunscreens

Both mineral and chemical sunscreens protect the skin from harmful UV radiation, but they differ both in their active ingredients and how they work. Here's a comparison of the two types:

Mineral sunscreens

Active ingredients:
- Zinc oxide
- Titanium dioxide
- Iron oxide

Mechanism:
- Physical barrier: mineral sunscreens sit on the skin's surface and reflect or scatter UV rays, preventing them from penetrating the skin.

Advantages:
- Starts working immediately upon application
- Broad-spectrum protection
- Gentle on skin
- Less likely to degrade in sunlight compared with certain chemical filters

Disadvantages:
- Mineral sunscreen tends to go on thick and white. It can be difficult to rub in, and it often leaves a white cast or chalky residue.

Chemical sunscreens

Active ingredients:
- Oxybenzone
- Avobenzone

- Octocrylene
- Octinoxate
- Homosalate
- Octisalate
- Other chemical compounds

Mechanism:
- Chemical absorption: absorbs UV radiation and converts it to heat, which is then released from the skin.

Advantages:
- Easy to apply and blend into the skin without leaving a white residue
- Often more water-resistant than mineral sunscreens
- Comes in a variety of formulations including sprays, lotions, and gels

Disadvantages:
- Higher potential for skin irritation, allergic reactions, and stinging, especially around the eyes
- Requires about 15 to 30 minutes to become effective after application
- Certain chemical ingredients, such as oxybenzone and octinoxate, have been listed to harm coral reefs; however, reef-safe sunscreens are available.

IR and HEV protection

The vast majority of sunscreens on the market today do not protect against IR or HEV, and any methods of defense against these types of rays are not regulated by the FDA. As a consumer, the best thing you can do is look for reputable brands that invest in clinical research and have high-quality, medical-grade ingredients. Sunscreens designed to protect against IR often contain antioxidants such as niacinamide and/or vitamins C and E, which neutralize the free radicals produced by IR exposure. Sunscreens designed to protect against HEV light often contain ingredients such as iron oxides, titanium dioxide, and specific antioxidants. These ingredients help shield the skin from the harmful effects of blue light.

You might be wondering whether everyone needs to be thinking about IR and HEV protection. The truth is that some need to worry about it more than others do. Pilots, who work at higher altitudes, and other individuals employed in the field of transportation should have daily protection against IR rays. With the boom in technology and more people spending all day in front of screens, protection against blue light also has become a major focus.

A note about iron oxide

This ingredient is used in tinted sunscreens, which contain pigments. It has a greater protective effect against blue light and is recommended for pigmentary disorders such as melasma in patients with darker skin tones.[38] However, iron oxides are the same pigments that are present in any foundation. In sunscreen, they have simply been encapsulated so that in iron-oxide sunscreens they appear to match your skin.

Safety concerns with chemicals

We're living in a time when the consumer zeitgeist is shifting to all-natural products, organic everything, local ingredients, and actually being able to pronounce and understand everything on a label. Overall, this is an overwhelmingly positive change in thinking—and it will help many industries move in a more positive direction to better protect people's health.

But when it comes to sunscreen, this change is leaving many people confused. If you've ever scrolled through the world of skincare on Tik-Tok, you've probably seen people questioning the safety of chemical sunscreens. Many have gone so far as to proclaim that there's no real benefit from sunscreen and that it's been thrust on us by big business seeking a profit.

As the world becomes more conscious of the harmful chemicals that people are exposed to on a daily basis, it's only natural to examine sunscreen as well. However, it's important to remember that sunscreen is different from other products because its sole purpose is to protect against a known danger: if you don't have sun protection, you are more likely to get cancer and die. You can't say the same thing about crackers, shampoo, or scented candles. Exposing yourself to the chemicals that are in many of those products/brands, even in small quantities, might not be worth it. But you can't forgo sun protection without drastically increasing your risk for the very thing it's designed to protect you against.

The safety of chemicals in sunscreens has been a topic of considerable debate and research for many years, and so far, the findings have been reassuring. For example, some studies suggest that oxybenzone, octinoxate, and homosalate may act as endocrine disruptors, mimicking or interfering with hormone function. Endocrine disruptors have been linked to a variety of health issues including reproductive problems, birth defects, and cancer. As a headline, this sounds terrible! However, when you dig into the details of these studies, the effects have primarily been observed in laboratory settings or animal studies at doses much higher than typical human exposure. The amount of any substance that goes into the bloodstream is a fraction of 1 percent. Newer formulations are designed to not get into the bloodstream.[39, 40]

Compare that with UV radiation, a known carcinogen that kills thousands of people every year. The proven benefits of sunscreens in preventing skin cancer far outweigh the potential risks associated with their ingredients.

Even if you're doing your best to avoid chemicals across the board, I urge you to consider making an exception when it comes to chemical sunscreen. If you're not open to doing that, you'll need to put in extra effort with mineral sunscreens and other methods of sun protection.

Proper application

Proper application is crucial in order for sunscreen to be effective. It should be applied generously and evenly to all exposed skin about 15 minutes before sun exposure. It should be reapplied every two hours, or more often if you have fair skin, or if you're swimming, sweating, or toweling off. Some sunscreens are labeled as water-resistant, meaning they provide protection while swimming or sweating for a specified time. However, water-resistant does not mean waterproof, and reapplication is necessary after swimming or excessive sweating.

Other options for sun protection

Broad-spectrum high-SPF sunscreen is essential, but it's still only part of a comprehensive sun-protection strategy.

- Shade: I'm saying it again because that's how important it is!
- Sunglasses: In addition to protecting your eyes (including safeguarding against macular degeneration later in life), sunglasses prevent you from squinting. This can help you stave off wrinkles around your eyes and make your Botox last longer.
- Hats: A baseball cap, or even better, a broad-brimmed hat, is a must for prolonged periods in the sun, especially if you're near water or sand. It not only protects your face from harmful rays, but it shields your eyes so you don't squint as much. (For maximum benefit, wear sunglasses and a hat!)
- Sun-protective clothing: Tightly woven fabrics are best for sun protection. You can also buy clothing with SPF protection built in. Another cost-effective way to protect yourself is with an inexpensive powder that washes into an entire load of laundry to provide a universal protection factor to clothes for up to 20 washes. Use this powder regularly to maintain ongoing protection.
- Polypodium leucotomos: Mentioned in the previous chapter, this daily supplement adds another layer of protection from harmful UV rays.
- Avoid tanning beds and booths: This should go without saying, but I'll mention it just in case anyone's beauty routine is still stuck in the 1980s. There are some great sunless tanning products on the market these days, so try those instead.
- Stay inside when the UV index is high: Check the report to see how much UV radiation is expected to reach the Earth's surface for your geographic area.

Get your skin checked!

I've lost track of how many of my patients have come in over the years for aesthetic treatments and left with a cancer diagnosis. The vast majority were saved with early detection. We even had one of these patients in our practice speak at Made for Shade this year.

If you're an aesthetic practitioner, consider it your duty to keep an eye out for skin cancer. There are hundreds of thousands of people out there right now who have skin cancer and don't know it. Though it's incredibly rewarding to help patients look their best through treatments, it pales in comparison to saving someone's life by catching skin cancer. I encourage you to lean into this opportunity and help as many people as you can.

And if you ever notice anything unusual happening with your skin, such as a new mole, bump, or growth that doesn't go away, or itches or changes to an existing mole, make an appointment with a board-certified dermatologist. Check the guide at the end of this book for signs to be aware of. You should also see a dermatologist at least once a year to have a preventative full-body scan. More than two people die of skin cancer in the United States every hour.[41] Early detection saves lives.

CHAPTER 6

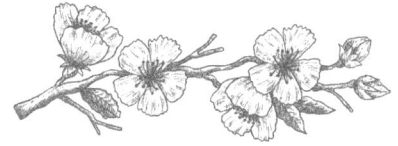

Step Up Your Skincare Routine

People have been creating skincare products for thousands of years, largely through trial and error. Some of those ingredients are still used in products today, whereas others are not.

A popular ingredient in European cosmetics from the 16th through 19th centuries was, perhaps shockingly, lead. Back then, women wanted their skin to look much like women do today: youthful. Skin becomes less reflective and lacks glow as people age, and more reflective skin is associated with a youthful complexion. Certain ingredients, such as lead, have properties that increase the amount of light reflecting off the skin, giving a luminous dewy complexion. The way these products make light scatter off a rough surface can also mask blemishes and imperfections.

Lead was tested recently as foundation on ethically sourced pigskin. The results were surprisingly similar to modern skincare products and foundations: skin looked smoother and more youthful.[42]

Today, we're still in hot pursuit of products that provide that youthful glow of good health—just without the poison. There are a variety of options for the face and body that work wonders for improving skin texture, elasticity, and glow. In this chapter, I share my best secrets for what really makes a noticeable difference in your skincare routine—and what's not worth the money.

Daily skincare routine for the face

There is a complex, 18-step skincare routine that certain Korean beauty enthusiasts swear by—and if you have the interest, time, and money for all that, more power to you! However, more is not always better. The four- to five-step skincare routine highlighted in this chapter more than adequately covers what the vast majority of people need. There are also opportunities to expand on these steps with additional products if you so choose.

Order: It's important to follow the steps in the order below or else some of the products might cancel out the effects of other products. If you wear makeup, apply it only after step 5.

Time: This routine is best performed both morning and night, and the products you use will be slightly different.

- Step 1: Wash
- Step 2: Apply growth factor (optional)
- Step 3: Add anything corrective
- Step 4: Moisturize and hydrate
- Step 5: Apply sunscreen (morning only)

Step 1: Wash

Your skin will look better and stay healthier if you wash your face twice per day. Most people should use a gentle cleanser that doesn't have drying ingredients. (If you live in a dry climate or you spend time in dry ambient air, it's especially important that you avoid ingredients that could sap more moisture from your skin.) If you have acne, an inflammatory skin condition, or signs of aging, then a medicated wash can be beneficial. In this case, look for products with salicylic acid, which is a beta-hydroxy acid (BHA) that helps clean out your pores by

A quick note on brands

More-expensive brands are not necessarily better. It's true that some luxury brands are worth the investment, but many rely more on marketing than quality. Here are a few basic distinctions between them:
- Prescription: If you have serious, specific skincare needs, a dermatologist can prescribe products that fit your needs.
- Medical grade: It's important to note that companies can use this term without following specific guidelines, but the general expectation here is that the company has invested in a significant amount of scientific research to ensure that their products actually work. This means that if they say a product does a specific thing, such as reduce the appearance of fine lines by 20 percent, there should be a reputable study to back that claim. Make sure they have gone through clinical trials, peer-reviewed journal publications, and studies on final formulations. If the products meet this burden, then true medical-grade products tend to be the most effective—but also the priciest.
- Over the counter: This is 90 percent of what's out there—whether it's a high-end or drugstore brand. Many of these companies frequently make claims that have no scientific backing. To avoid wasting your money or time using a product that doesn't work, you generally want to go for national brands that are specifically known for skincare, have been around a while, and are well respected.

reaching deep into them and breaking down bonds between keratinocytes. Alpha-hydroxy acids, also known as AHAs, are a group of acids found in fruits, sugarcane, and milk. Examples include lactic acid (dairy and fermented vegetables), glycolic acid (sugarcane), malic acid (apples), citric acid (citrus fruits), and tartaric acid (grapes). They help improve skin texture while reducing the visible signs of aging, hyperpigmentation, melasma, acne, and sun damage.

Whether you opt for a gentle face wash or a medicated wash, lukewarm water is best, as hot water can remove the skin's protective oils. Use your bare hands instead of a washcloth. When you're finished washing, gently pat dry with a towel instead of rubbing at your skin.

And while you're at it, don't forget to wash your hair regularly! Patients come into my office all the time with pityrosporum folliculitis, which are little waxy bumps around their hairline, and they think it's acne or some kind of a rash when it's usually yeast buildup from dirty hair. Hot and humid climates and/or excessive sweating can make this condition worse. If you experience this, you might want to try a medicated shampoo with selenium sulfide, or a topical ketoconazole.

To exfoliate or not to exfoliate?

That is the question many people are wondering. And for good reason! Though there are thousands of exfoliators on the market, in reality, it's not a type of product that everyone actually needs. You grow a new layer of skin every month. If it's healthy, you don't need to scrub it off before it sheds naturally—especially when it comes to the delicate skin on your face, neck, and chest.

That said, certain conditions can be improved by exfoliation, such as getting rid of sebaceous filaments, the black spots usually found on the nose that are often confused with blackheads. Another situation that might call for exfoliation (or an ablative laser) is keratosis pilaris, the bumpy "chicken skin" on the upper arms. (Most people get this when they're young and eventually outgrow it.)

If you think your skin is rough and you want to exfoliate gently, you can use products with alphaor beta-hydroxy acids, such as glycolic acid, lactic acid, mandelic acid, citric acid, or malic acid. Note that you do not need a grainy product to scrape the bumps off your skin.

Toner

As a teenager in the 1980s, I definitely used toner. However, this is not something we were trained to use in dermatology. Welcome to the 2000s; it's beyond time you tossed your toner.

Step 2: Apply growth factor (optional)

Growth factors play an important role in keeping other cells alive and healthy as they communicate essential messages between cells to promote healing and growth. We all have natural growth-factor cells, but as we age, our production decreases, reducing our skin's ability to maintain elasticity and firmness. Many products on the market contain growth factors, and they have many sources from which they are derived.

This is an area where science has come a long way! After years of research, we're finally able to pinpoint ingredients that have been clinically proven to make a difference in reducing fine lines and wrinkles and improving skin tone and texture. These ingredients come from every corner of the world and include hundreds of botanicals, marine extracts, and peptides. For instance, some sources include human neonatal fibroblast tissue, recombinant plants, bone derivation, mesenchyme, snails—the list goes on.[43] Skincare companies create special proprietary blends of these growth factors and package them in a variety of ways. They aren't usually specifically labeled as growth factors—likely because most consumers don't know what that means. Instead, products are usually labeled with messaging such as anti-aging, skin rejuvenation, healing and repair, advanced technology, or having a high concentration of specific ingredients such as green tea, plankton extract, or algae.

Like all skincare products, some work much better than others—and there is a huge range in price points. The ones that have been clinically proven to work and are made by companies that invest a lot of money in research and are therefore often quite expensive. In fact, if you choose to incorporate this step into your skincare routine, it will likely be the most expensive product on your shelf.

In terms of effectiveness, the cause or origin of the growth factor is what matters most. As humans, our tissue is most responsive to human neonatal fibroblast tissue because this growth factor fits into our cells with a perfect key-lock configuration. Other sources may help to increase collagen levels, elastin, and other factors, but currently, nothing is superior to human neonatal fibroblast tissue.[44]

My favorite skincare brand is SkinMedica because they've done such an incredible job researching ingredients that make a real difference in skin health and appearance and creating products that truly work. That said, they are certainly a high-end brand, and their products can be considered a splurge. If you want to go this route and use a growth-factor product with neonatal fibroblast tissue, my favorite products are the TNS Advanced + Serum and the TNS Recovery Complex.[45] Though they are expensive, I've found them to make a noticeable difference. In fact, this splurge can average out to be a value since it is so effective.

Other types of growth factors have become quite popular in recent years as well, including mucin powder. When it's derived from snail mucin (snail secretion filtrate), it offers numerous skincare benefits, including hydration and the reduction of fine lines and wrinkles. High-potency mucin powder is expensive. It works—but not as well as either TNS product. In fact, according to a study in the *Journal of Drugs in Dermatology* in 2017, TNS products—even the older versions—work twice as well as snail mucin powder. Also, lower-cost mucin powder is also lower in potency, which means it's even less effective.

A different product that has the white papers to show its efficacy is the Revision DEJ Daily Boosting Serum.[46] This novel approach is based on the power of sunflower seeds. If I had to choose a product behind either of the TNS products, it would be this one.

This step is an area where you want to make sure you aren't spending money on products that don't make a noticeable difference. I often have reps from various companies reach out to me to discuss their products. The difference is in the white papers. Don't be fooled by pretty marketing or by the companies that tell you that their clinical trials are better. Have them show you the clinical trials and the studies on final formulation for their products; whenever products are proven to make a real difference, there will be at least one published peer-reviewed journal research paper saying so. If neither the splurge brand or high-potency mucin powder is in your reach, then I recommend going with a reliable national brand and applying a serum rather than a growth factor. Neutrogena, CeraVe, or Cetaphil are all good choices.

Step 3: Add anything corrective

This skincare step can be executed in a variety of ways. The idea is to treat specific issues that concern you.

Don't forget your neck and chest

When it comes to steps 3 through 5, don't forget your neck and chest! This skin is similar to your face in that it's a focal point on your body, relatively thin, and highly susceptible to wrinkles.

Skin-tone-evening products

Skin-tone-evening products work by targeting various factors that contribute to uneven skin tone, such as hyperpigmentation, dark spots, redness, and dullness. Many include brightening agents and antioxidants. Achieving more-even skin tone typically requires consistent use of these products over time. Results may vary depending on individual skin type, the severity of the pigmentation issues, and adherence to your skincare routine.

For patients who are considering aesthetic treatments to create a more-even skin tone, using topical products is generally a good place to start. After a few months of diligent use, doing so can often provide a better starting point for other treatments. And of course, don't forget how important sun protection is for evening the skin tone. Wearing sunscreen and hats will truly make a difference to your skin's appearance.

Retinol products: Retinol is a form of vitamin A that is used in skincare products for various benefits. It's most commonly used as an anti-aging product due to its ability to reduce the appearance of fine lines, wrinkles, and age spots, but it can also be effective for treating acne, particularly in the prescription form as a retinoid. Retinol works by increasing the rate of normal cell production and skin turnover. It can cause irritation and drying and should be introduced only gradually to your skincare routine. To maximize effectiveness, wait 30 minutes after washing your face before you apply retinol. This step should only be done at night since retinol can become less effective in sunlight.

Niacinamide: Niacin supports your body on a cellular level and is involved in DNA repair and synthesis. Niacinamide enhances the production of ceramides, which are lipid molecules that form a crucial part of the skin barrier. It strengthens the skin's natural barrier, helping to retain moisture and protect against environmental irritants and pollutants. Niacinamide has anti-inflammatory properties that can help calm irritated skin, making it beneficial for conditions such as acne, rosacea, and eczema, reducing redness and inflammation.[47]

There's also a study that shows a decrease in skin cancers from using niacinamide orally, so don't forget to take your vitamins.[48]

Brightening products

Brightening products are skincare formulations that are designed to improve the radiance and luminosity of the skin, typically by targeting dullness, uneven skin tone, and dark spots. Brighteners can work by inhibiting melanin production (which causes those dark spots) and promoting a more-even distribution of pigment in the skin. Ingredients such as vitamin C, niacinamide (vitamin B3), licorice extract, and arbutin are known for their brightening properties.

Lotus-sprout extract: This is one of the ingredients I'm most excited about! SkinMedica has put a large amount of research into lotus-sprout extract, and the findings are inspiring, as evidenced by its Even and Correct product line, which the company discovered with in-silico production. Lotus-sprout extract is rich in antioxidants, so it protects the skin from free-radical damage and environmental stressors. Its anti-inflammatory properties soothe irritation and reduce redness, while its hydrating effects keep the skin plump and moisturized. The extract also brightens your complexion, reducing dark spots and hyperpigmentation, and promotes cell regeneration, helping to diminish fine lines and wrinkles. Additionally, lotus-sprout extract detoxifies the skin, removing impurities and promoting a clearer, healthier appearance. I imagine we'll be seeing this ingredient in a lot of products in the future!

Vitamin C and antioxidants

Vitamin C offers multiple skin benefits, making it a popular skincare ingredient. As a powerful antioxidant, it protects the skin from free radicals and environmental stressors such as UV rays and pollution. It boosts collagen production, essential for maintaining skin elasticity and firmness, reducing fine lines and wrinkles. Vitamin C also helps even skin tone by lightening hyperpigmentation and brown spots, leading to a brighter complexion. Its anti-inflammatory properties reduce redness and irritation, which are particularly beneficial for acne-prone skin. Additionally, it enhances the skin's natural healing process and boosts the efficacy of sunscreen, providing comprehensive protection and improvement for overall skin health. Some of my favorite vitamin C products are by Revision with its C+ Correcting Complex and new C+ Brightening Eye Complex.[49]

Vitamin C can work well for a lot of people; however, it can also cause skin irritation. If you've experienced this, or you're interested in trying other antioxidants, there are several great options on the market.

My respected dermatology colleague Dr. Jacqueline Calkin has a thriving practice in Sacramento, and she loves the SkinCeuticals line. Her go-to product is CE Ferulic, which she considers the original antioxidant. She respects the company's clinical studies on effectiveness and that the product can be layered with other products. She's also noticed that many of her male patients can get on board with it if they want to use only one thing. Her patients report that it works, and they appear to love it.

Dr. Calkin also recommends SkinCeuticals P-TIOX Serum, which is a new neuropeptide-based product that gives the quickest results she has ever seen. "Once people start it, they want to keep using it," she says. "It helps people achieve glass skin and minimizes expression lines that can't be treated with Botox."

The Lumivive system from SkinMedica is one of my favorites. In fact, I think it's the biggest secret on the market for skin rejuvenation. It has a Nobel Prize–winning formulation that uses the skin's circadian rhythm to restore skin health. There's one product for the daytime and another for the evening, and they work in different ways. Water loss and cell repair are greatest in the nighttime, and it's important to capitalize on this factor and maintain intrinsic health. That's why the nighttime product uses next-generation mitoquinol mesylate that gets into the cells and helps to feed ATP.[50] Since we lose the ability to repair our cells as we age and our body has a difficult time incorporating energy ATP into our cells, this work-around is brilliant. Think of all that time while you're asleep: it is your body's time to repair and revitalize. However, with age, that efficiency fades. For this reason, Lumivive doesn't just address how your skin looks, as after 12 weeks of use, your skin's cancer markers will have decreased. To prove this claim, SkinMedica used a third-party facility in France to conduct the research, and when the results came out, it was a big deal. Unfortunately, however, that news was quickly overshadowed by the outbreak of COVID-19. I don't think that many people in the organization, outside the research group at least, even know that much about it. I hope the company can become louder about this anti-cancer evidence—and that the FDA allows it to do so.

During the day, extrinsic aging occurs and we are pelted with pollution, ionizing radiation, and other external factors that can age us. This is when people traditionally grab their vitamin C serum. However, what I respect about the daytime Lumivive system is that it is next level and "not your mother's vitamin C" as it uses non-irritating ingredients to protect skin from cancer-causing agents.[51] SkinMedica even studied this product on other continents, including one of the most polluted cities in the world, New Delhi. The results show that outdoor workers who wore it had a decrease in cancer-causing free radicals on their skin. I can't emphasize enough how superior this is to traditional vitamin C because not only is it an antioxidant, but it also decreases cancer markers on the skin. I like to think of this as a dual agent that not only prevents but also reverses cancer.

Neck creams: Much like eye creams, there are certainly high-quality products on the market that are designed specifically to treat the skin on your neck. If you have the interest and budget to add this to your skincare routine, you might enjoy the results. Another way to look at this is by seeing your neck as an extension of your face and applying the same corrective or moisturizing products to this part of your body. Alternately, if your skin is on the drier side, you might want to use body lotion on your neck, especially when the weather is cold or dry. This is likely to be much less expensive, and you'll still get the primary benefit: moisturizing power.

If you are struggling with excess adipose (fat) tissue in this area, there are products on the market that claim to be beneficial for this. Check out Nectifirm Advanced by Revision.[52] However, if it's more of a chicken-skin appearance in this area that is concerning you, then a cream with an agent to address this would be most beneficial. I like Neck Correct by SkinMedica for this issue. The medicinal herb paracress ingredient works to stop the arrector-pili muscles from contracting and makes the hair follicles and surrounding atrophic/thinned skin less noticeable.[53]

Step 4: Moisturize and hydrate

One of the easiest things anyone can do to make their skin healthier and look better is to properly moisturize. My nurses will tell you that this is one of my biggest teaching points in my clinic. Chronic dryness can accelerate the aging process by contributing to the appearance of fine lines and wrinkles, making the skin look older than it is. This happens because dry skin lacks the necessary moisture to maintain its elasticity and resilience. Further, skin loses its moisture as we age, so it becomes even more important to diligently moisturize.

Aesthetic treatments can help improve the skin's quality and appearance, but when a person doesn't keep up with proper moisturizing, many treatments don't work as well as they would otherwise, or last as long.

Some of my favorite moisturizers are CeraVe Moisturizing Cream, Cetaphil Moisturizing Cream, Neutrogena Hydro Boost Body Gel Cream, and Curel Hydra Therapy Wet Skin Moisturizer.

I hold fast to my dermatology roots when it comes to oils. The American Academy of Dermatology (AAD) does not recommend them for several reasons: they tend to not soak in as well, can be comedogenic (pore-clogging), and can be a slip-and-fall hazard in the bathroom. (That last one might make you chuckle, but it's a real concern when people are wet out of the shower.)

Hyaluronic acid: Hyaluronic acid is a naturally occurring substance in the body and is known for its remarkable ability to retain moisture. It can hold up to 1,000 times its weight in water, making it highly effective at maintaining moisture levels in the skin. And as you know by now, keeping skin hydrated is the key for improving skin health and appearance, including upholding elasticity and staving off fine lines and wrinkles.

My favorite hack from this section is to use hyaluronic acid with moist fingertips and pat onto the skin, especially around my eyes. I recommend the newly launched hyaluronic acid from SkinMedica. Yes, I love SkinMedica—but it's the science I love the most. And wet fingertips are no longer a requirement with its new Hydra Collagen HA5.

There are other quality hyaluronic acids available in beauty stores and drugstores, such as ISDIN Hyaluronic Concentrate, La Roche-Posay Hyalu B5 Pure, and Neutrogena Hydro Boost.

HA5 from SkinMedica has been proven to decrease the appearance of wrinkles within 15 minutes, and then in 16 hours, it increases the body's ability to create its own hyaluronic acid. At my practice, we apply it after Botox. It's a nice little extra boost with immediate gratification on the results. We got this hack from a study done by Sabrina Fabi, MD, FAAD.[54]

Eye creams: A lot of people wonder whether eye cream is a scam given how it is one of the more expensive skincare products available. Here's my take on it. The skin is a little different around the eyes since that's where it's the thinnest on the body. Too many chemicals aren't good because the skin is a bit more sensitive than in other areas. There are wonderful eye creams out there that work to keep skin moisturized and healthy; however, you don't need a product that's specific for this part of the body. Try a gentle creamy moisturizer that is noncomedogenic, which means it won't clog pores. For a splurge, try the new C+ Brightening Eye Complex by Revision mentioned previously.[55]

Gold: Who doesn't love a little gold? The gold-infused eye hydrogel eye mask from NakedBeauty MD is a hot new product. I met the inventor, Dr. Catherine Chang, when we were on an ad board together in West Hollywood. I enjoy following her on Instagram for her skincare advice.

Step 5: Apply sunscreen (morning only)

This step is so important that I covered it at length in the previous chapter. You should be wearing sunscreen every day, and whatever amount of it comes already mixed into your foundation cannot be relied upon as your only sunscreen. After reading the last chapter, you probably know why! Foundation usually says something like "SPF 30," and it's rarely labeled as broad spectrum. Even if it were, most makeup brands don't focus on sunscreen, and the sun protection their products offer is likely inferior to actual high-quality sunscreen.

Iron oxide: For people with olive or darker skin tone who have melasma, iron oxide provides extra sun protection. This can be found in sunscreen and is one of the essential pigments in foundation. For shade-matching sunscreen, the pigment is usually encapsulated and, when rubbed in, bursts and appears to match your skin tone.

Best practices for products

Test your products

Before you apply a new product to your face, it's smart to test it somewhere else on your body in case you have a reaction. I recommend testing products on your inner elbow for three consecutive nights. In dermatology, we call this the "poor man's patch test." If an adverse reaction occurs, stop using the product. To treat irritated skin or patch-test-positive skin, a 1-percent hydrocortisone cream can be used up to 14 days per month—and you can combine it with an antihistamine daily as needed. And here's a hot tip: many skincare stores will let you return products for free if they give you a bad reaction, so make sure you look into that!

Should you leave skincare products in the fridge?

Cute little skincare refrigerators have become all the rage—especially for teens and tweens who are obsessed with skincare. But does it really matter whether you keep your beauty products cold? This trend likely started because certain products, including compounded medications such as benzoyl peroxide, stay stable longer in the fridge. Always check the recommended storage temperature on a product before you choose your storage tactic; the vast majority of other products don't need this kind of special treatment. As long as you're keeping products at room temperature rather than in a hot car, you should be good to go. (That said, if it makes you feel fancy to keep your face cream in a little pink fridge on your vanity, do it!)

How long do products last?

Check the packaging and you'll find a version of an expiration date that usually relates to how long a product stays good after it's been opened.

For example, "12M" suggests that the quality can be relied on for 12 months after opening. Generally speaking, if products are stored at their recommended temperature, they are good for much longer than the date listed on the product.

Personally, I tend not to focus too much on expiration dates for non-medicated topical products. I'll go ahead and use them, and whenever I determine that they aren't effective anymore, I toss them out and buy something new.

Periodic treatments for the face
Facials

Facials can be an excellent way to boost skin health periodically throughout the year. They help maintain clear pores, promote cell turnover, and keep the skin balanced and hydrated. A number of my patients love to schedule a facial a few days before a wedding, party, or other significant event to give their skin a healthy, radiant glow. Facials can also be great for treating acne.

However, there are certain patients who shouldn't have facials, particularly those with sensitive skin, rosacea, and/or allergies. It makes me cringe when I see a spa offering a "rosacea facial." Please take these off your list of services!

Diamond Glow

This facial treatment by SkinMedica is a pen-like microdermabrasion instrument that gently removes the top layer of skin. It exfoliates, deeply cleanses pores, and infuses skin with a powerful serum. The serum contains many of the ingredients I highlighted for daily skincare, including growth factors, hyaluronic acids, and brightening agents such as lotus-sprout-derived Even and Correct. With Diamond Glow, these ingredients penetrate deeper into the skin and have more staying power.

Within 72 hours, most people experience a visible improvement to the appearance of fine lines, radiance, and hydration. The benefits continue to last up to 12 weeks, when people often experience improvement in hyperpigmentation, photodamage repair, skin-tone evenness, and texture.

I love the results of Diamond Glow, and so do my patients. At my clinic, it's one of our most popular facial treatments. The results speak for themselves, and the treatment is relaxing and enjoyable.

Dermaplaning

This is a minimally invasive method of removing dead skin cells to smooth and brighten skin and remove the fine baby fuzz from the face. Dermaplaning can also reduce the appearance of acne scars and soften fine lines and wrinkles. Recommended frequency is about four to six weeks. Dermaplaning can make skin sensitive, so it's always good to do this with caution so that you don't damage your skin or irritate it. Most people can use a gentle version of this at home or as an add-on to microdermabrasion at a clinic.

Latisse

Having longer, thicker eyelashes can do a lot for making eyes seem brighter and giving a more youthful appearance. Latisse works well for most people. Writing a prescription for patients can be an easy way to drive results they'll love.

Daily skincare routine for the body

Moisturizer

It's helpful to think of the skin envelope as a sealed barrier. When it's dry, it has microscopic holes where bacteria and irritants can get in and moisture gets out. This can cause a whole range of health issues, including increasing the risk of infection. The goal is to keep the whole skin envelope properly sealed by maintaining a high level of moisture. This is an area where many people try but fall short!

I like to use the mantra "soak and seal." After a shower, the skin is most hydrated due to the absorption of water. (Washing your face in the sink doesn't necessarily have the same effect since it's a much quicker and less-steamy process than a shower.) Applying body lotion immediately after bathing helps to lock in moisture, preventing the skin from evaporating and keeping it hydrated longer. Additionally, the skin's permeability is higher when it is damp, meaning that it can more effectively absorb the active ingredients in moisturizers, thereby ensuring that the skin gets the maximum benefit from the product.

Lotion should be applied all over the entire body wherever you can reach. Hands, elbows, legs, and feet tend to get especially dry. Applying once a day might be enough for some parts of your body, depending on your geography and the time of year. Most people should be applying moisturizer to their hands multiple times a day, especially if you wash them often.

The type of product you use makes a huge difference in your results. In fact, your body lotion might be making your skin even more dry if the water content is higher than the humidity level in the ambient air. When this happens, lotion will evaporate and pull even more water out of your skin. So if you live in Arizona and you apply a thin, watery body lotion, chances are that you're left feeling pretty dry. You might be thinking it's unavoidable because of the climate, but what you really need is an especially thick, creamy moisturizer to coat your skin and help lock in moisture.

Most lotions are petroleum based, with water and alcohol added to make the product thinner. From there, they get whipped, much like egg whites. The longer the product is whipped, the creamier it gets. If you live in a dry climate, you want a product that will form stiff peaks. (Anything that comes out in a pump is too watery.) If you live in a tropical environment, most of the time, a thinner moisturizer is going to be just fine.

Make sure you avoid the slippery slope of having skin get so dry that it becomes itchy, flaky, and difficult to treat. This can easily lead to other skin conditions, such as eczema, that might require medical treatment and prescription medication.

You don't need to buy anything fancy or expensive to keep your skin hydrated, although there are plenty of products out there that contain some of the same superpower ingredients and growth factors you find in moisturizers and serums marketed for the face. If you're at all conscious of your budget, this is an area where you might not want to invest too much, since your money will go further with higher-quality products for your face.

Try these products (listed in order from thinnest to thickest):

- Curel Hydra Therapy Wet Skin Moisturizer (Apply it in the shower after you turn the water off. Then get out and pat dry with a towel. It's clinically proven to hydrate skin.)
- Neutrogena Hydro Boost Body Gel Cream
- Cetaphil Moisturizing Cream
- CeraVe Moisturizing Cream (especially the one that comes in a jar)
- Vanicream (This is made by the Mayo Clinic and is especially good for people with sensitive skin.)
- Eucerin cream
- Aquaphor or Vaseline/petroleum jelly for a thicker barrier

Firming products

Some areas of the body can benefit from a little firming and tightening, and there are a number of products that are effective in reducing the appearance of flabbiness, creepiness, and/or cellulite. My favorite product is Firm and Tone from SkinMedica. A recent study shows that it stimulates the dermal extracellular matrix and improves cellulite and sagging. I've seen the results myself after using it on my own body! It's on the pricier side, so I save it for my arms and legs, where I most want to firm and decrease the appearance of cellulite. If you want to try another brand that's less expensive, look for products that contain caffeine, which is an effective ingredient.

Compression socks

A lot of people suffer from spider and varicose veins. There are aesthetic treatments for improving the appearance of these conditions, but it's often easier to prevent them than treat them later. Compression socks work wonders for providing graduated pressure to the legs, which improves blood flow and reduces venous pressure. By pushing blood upward against gravity and toward the heart, blood pooling is prevented and veins don't become visible.

Compression socks are recommended for whenever you spend prolonged periods of time sitting or standing, such as long flights or road trips. I wear them every day that I'm working, since I spend so much time on my feet seeing patients. I like to joke with my patients that I have been wearing compression socks for more than 20 years—just not the same pair! They're also great during pregnancy, as pregnant women often experience increased swelling and are at higher risk of developing varicose veins due to hormonal changes and increased blood volume.

Another great trick to get the blood flowing away from your feet and reduce swelling after a long day is to lie down somewhere you can put your feet up against a wall. Stay in that position for about 10 minutes and you should feel a difference. You can also tell your family that you are exercising if they see you lying there. This usually gets a nice eyeroll in my home!

When it comes to skincare, the earlier you develop a good routine, the better. By regular use of high-quality products, you can extend the youthfulness of your skin by years—if not a decade or more. It's one of those things that takes extra effort and doesn't necessarily drive immediate results, but it's well worth it.

If you're an aesthetic practitioner, make sure your patients are doing everything within their power and budget to take care of their skin properly at home. This will decrease their need for aesthetic treatments, which is a good thing!

CHAPTER 7

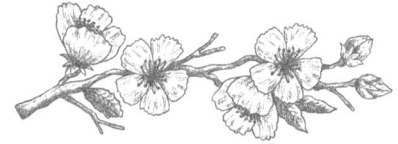

Light and Lasers

Most people who know me—professionally or personally—know that I love laser treatments. I'm a proponent of all different kinds of aesthetic treatments, but lasers are by far my favorite. I think they are the most underrated aesthetic service and often the best option for achieving the outcomes that people want. Oftentimes, when patients come in thinking they want Botox, or filler, or microneedling, they would get better results by doing a laser treatment before or instead of those other options.

But if you would have asked me about lasers in 1997, I would have told you something completely different. I was in med school that year doing my rounds through various specialties, and one day still sticks out in my mind decades later as being especially impactful.

I was doing a plastic-surgery rotation, and a patient came in to have C_{O2} laser resurfacing on her face for wrinkles. This procedure was a new experience for me, and I had never seen anything like it. The patient was in her 50s, and she was excited to look younger. Knowing that lasers could offer patients the aesthetic results they were looking for, I was excited for her too!

Back then, laser treatment was done in a hospital operating room, and anesthesiologists put patients under complete sedation. When our patient was asleep and resting comfortably, I remember looking at her and thinking she was in store for something truly exciting.

Laser in hand, the doctor began working on her face. Right away, I was surprised by how invasive it was. C_{O2} lasers are ablative, which means they physically cut the skin. Her wrinkles were definitely disappearing—but it was because her entire top layer of skin was disappearing. The next hour was one of the most difficult things I've ever had to watch. The doctor kept lasering and lasering until her face could only be described as a bloody pulp. My stomach turned, and I did everything in my power to appear calm and collected.

When the procedure was finally over, we put an ointment on what was left of the patient's face and wrapped her with Kerlix gauze tape like a mummy. She was taken to a recovery room, and I can only imagine what her loved one must have thought when they were reunited with her.

When an ablative laser goes that deep into the skin, it takes time for the body to heal. From there, her face would still be raw and bloody for about a week. It would take another week or so for new pink skin to form, and then a couple more weeks until she could go out in public without scaring the people around her. From there, her skin would continue healing over the course of several months, with new layers growing back and peeling off.

That's a long road to recovery for treating wrinkles!

On top of this, there was serious risk of scarring. Often, these patients have deeper wrinkles around their mouth, so the practitioner went deeper with their treatment in this area, and the effect was often a definitive hypopigmented ring around the mouth that differed from the surrounding tissue. There are also risks of scarring during the healing process due to inflammation caused by peeling or if the patient gets too much sun.

There's a whole generation of patients who got this lasering. These days, they're in their 70s, and I care for many of them in my dermatology practice. I can still tell which patients had this done by their light, shiny, pale skin around the mouth.

Lasers have come a long way since the 1990s. Today, we have nonablative lasers that work by using focused light to penetrate the skin and target various issues. On top of this, we also have red-light therapy and blue-light therapy, which use low-energy, broad-spectrum light to target superficial skin layers. I've seen firsthand how these treatments can provide a wide range of benefits that patients are looking for without intense pain or a long recovery time. I've seen lasers and light treatments do wonders for turning back skin damage, tightening skin, and helping people look significantly younger. They can correct uneven skin tone, get rid of birthmarks and scars, treat acne, help with rosacea, regrow hair, remove unwanted hair, make spider veins disappear, and "erase" tattoos. If aesthetic practitioners were magicians, lasers and light treatments could easily be considered our magic wands.

But the most remarkable thing about these services isn't that they improve physical appearance. It's the fact that they can reduce the likelihood of getting skin cancer. By removing damaged skin, lasers and light therapy can stimulate the production of new, healthy skin cells and collagen. This turnover reduces the likelihood of pre-cancerous cells returning or progressing into skin cancer.

Most people don't realize how much sun damage they actually have on their face and body. They think they have freckles, but those little brown marks are actually spots from sun damage. (Freckles go away in the winter. Dark marks that never go away are not freckles—no matter how cute they are.) These spots of damaged skin are more likely to turn into cancer than healthy skin. But it's not just about the spots we can see with the naked eye. For many people, the whole top layer of skin on their face, neck, and chest has the kind of damage that invites pre-cancerous cells to grow. Laser and light treatments remove this layer of skin, essentially turning back the clock for skin health. It doesn't get much closer to magic than that!

Lasers and light treatment are going through a renaissance right now. The advances in technology are incredible and leading to better and better outcomes. New lasers are high energy and rapid output, which means they penetrate the skin much faster than the previous generation of machines do. And because there are more points of contact with the machine, the laser doesn't need to penetrate as deeply to get the job done. That means less pain for the patient, a quicker treatment, and less recovery time.

Advances in technology have also made lasers significantly easier to use. For both practitioners and patients, this is a huge win. It used to require many hours of training and numerous procedures for practitioners to develop expertise in using lasers. Today, practitioners only need to use a machine a few times before becoming proficient at using it. That's because the lasers are largely controlled by computer. As you operate the laser, the computer tracks your speed and prevents you from going too slowly and burning the patient or too fast and potentially ending up with gap areas. With intelligent controls, you can do a person's entire back in minutes, as opposed to the 30 to 45 minutes it would take in years past.

Red-light therapy and blue-light therapy have gained significant popularity recently thanks to viral TikTok videos and new in-home devices. Before that, there was a bump in popularly in skincare during the early 2000s, but their actual development began much earlier. Red-light therapy was first researched by NASA in the 1990s to promote wound healing and tissue repair for astronauts in space. Funny enough, many of these studies were carried out by the Medical College of Wisconsin while I was in med school there![56] Around the same time, studies also found that both red and blue lights could be beneficial for skin health. By the mid-2000s, aesthetic practitioners started using light therapy to treat acne, reduce inflammation, and improve skin texture.

In this chapter, I cover what you need to know about using lasers and light treatments in order to get the best possible results.

First, let's get clear on the technology that is available today and what might cause you to choose certain options.

Lasers

Ablative vs. non-ablative:

- **Ablative lasers**: These are the original lasers in aesthetics (e.g., C_{O2} lasers, erbium lasers), and they remove the outer layers of skin. Note that though these are considered the "cutting" lasers, it's really more of a sandblasting device than a cutting mechanism. Rather than working with light, these lasers create controlled wounds on the outer-most layer of skin (or however deep the practitioner chooses to go), which leads to the formation of new skin cells as the skin heals. The chromophore for these lasers is water, rather than color, which means the wavelength is beyond the visible light spectrum.[57]

Wavelengths of light and the depth of penetration into the dermis

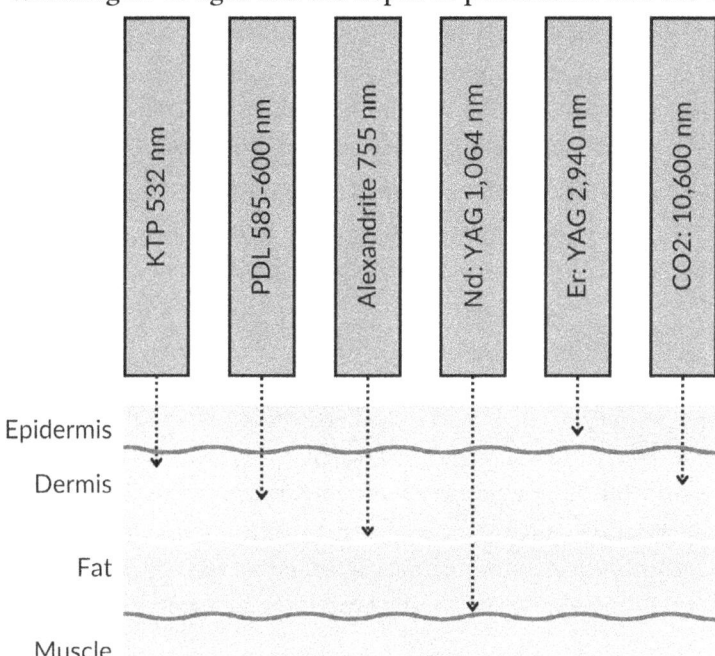

The bars in the chart from the left: KTP 532 nm, PDL 585-600 nm, Alexandrite 755 nm, Nd:YAG 1064 nm, Er:YAG 2940 nm, CO2 10,600 nm

- **Non-ablative lasers:** These lasers work beneath the surface of the skin without removing layers. Instead of cutting/sandblasting the top layer of skin, they operate underneath it by creating controlled thermal injury to the dermis, which triggers the skin's natural healing process and collagen production without damaging the epidermis. Non-ablative lasers can penetrate the skin at different depths, depending on the wave lengths used. The chromophore is not water but a color on the ROYGBIV spectrum—usually a shade of black, brown, red, etc. When the laser targets these colors, it helps treat issues within that color range. For example, targeting black or brown can remove hair of that color, and targeting red can treat rosacea or general collagen.

Mechanisms of action:

- **Selective photothermolysis:** Lasers work on the principle of selective photothermolysis, wherein the light energy is absorbed by the target tissue (e.g., melanin in dark spots or hemoglobin in blood vessels) without damaging surrounding tissue.
- **Heat generation:** The absorbed light from the laser gets converted to heat, which can destroy the target tissue, stimulate collagen production, or vaporize the outer layers of skin.

Types

There are a variety of lasers on the market worldwide, and they specialize in treating various conditions. A laser that is perfect for one person could create bad outcomes, or no outcomes at all, for another. And some laser machines are higher quality than others. This causes a great deal of confusion for patients, especially since marketing around laser treatments doesn't always specify the type or brand of equipment used by a practitioner.

Here are a few of the lasers I recommend for a variety of penetration levels into the dermis:

- **Broad-band laser (BBL):** This is the new version of the intense pulsed light (IPL) treatment. IPL uses light energy to target a certain color in your skin. When the skin is heated, your body gets rid of the unwanted cells, and that gets rid of the issue you're being treated for. It can treat a range of skin conditions at the same time. After IPL, you may look younger because your skin tone is more even. This laser is my go-to option as the least invasive treatment. I recommend a BBL for patients who want the gentlest option with the least amount of downtime. For patients who are in their 30s, or even their 40s, this might be all they need to improve minor signs of aging. This is a good maintenance laser treatment, and I recommend it once a year for many patients.
- **1,927 nanometer lasers, such as Moxi:** This is the next step up in terms of intensity for non-ablative laser. I use this laser when patients have a little more skin damage or haven't had a

laser treatment in quite a while and are looking for noticeable results, even if that means having more than a week of downtime. It operates on a wavelength of light of 1,927 nanometers (nm), and it works by essentially poking little aerated holes in the skin that are the equivalent thickness of two to two and a half sheets of paper. A Moxi laser treatment is generally something that is done on occasion, rather than regularly as maintenance. Though this type of laser can be used on all skin types, it might cause increased redness for type I (fair) skin. However, combining this procedure with a BBL during the same treatment time has been shown to help minimize the redness.

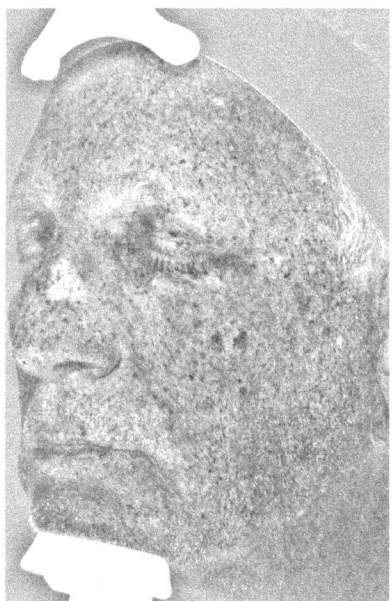

This 'before' image reveals areas of UV damage, porphyrins (bacteria), and brown spots on the skin. Advanced laser treatments like Moxi and BBL can help minimize pigmentation, smooth fine lines, refine texture, reduce pore size, and target redness—leaving your skin healthier and more radiant.

- **Fractional lasers, such as Halo:** A more recent invention, fractional lasers simultaneously deliver a non-ablative 1,470 nm and an ablative 2,940 nm wavelength to the same microscopic treatment zone, which creates an improvement in the appearance of aging skin. This is a more intense treatment since it has the combination of non-ablative and ablative laser. Its coverge is a little denser and goes two and a half to seven sheets of paper deep. This is generally a good option for patients who are in their 50s or older and show significant signs of aging.

- **C_{O2} lasers:** At 10,600 nm, this is the original ablative laser that many practices got started using, and a lot of them still have and use one regularly. It can be helpful when patients have deep wrinkles, scars, warts, or other severe skin issues. Proper anesthesia is important, as are sterility and strict adherence to post-wound care.

- **Erbium lasers (a.k.a. total resurfacing):** An erbium laser is a type of laser that uses targeted energy to remove damaged skin layers and treat a variety of skin conditions. It's also known as an erbium-YAG laser, which stands for erbium-doped yttrium aluminum garnet. With its 2,940 nm wavelength of light, erbium lasers—which are a nano laser and micro laser that, along with deep resurfacing, constitute "total resurfacing"—are similar to the old C_{O2} lasers but are a newer generation. They are ideal for severely photodamaged patients who have deeper lines and wrinkles that the less aggressive lasers can't get to. These lasers use erbium to target the water in skin cells, making them less aggressive than C_{O2} lasers. This is the best choice, in my opinion, for perioral wrinkles (fine or deep lines that appear around the mouth and lips). Be aware that these lasers can ablate down to several different depths, but the deepest they go in one pass is two sheets of paper, or as superficial as the stratum corneum.[58] The nano laser peel is 4 to 10 microns deep, the micro laser peel is 10 to 50 microns deep, and the deep resurfacing is 50 to 200 microns.

- **Pulsed dye lasers (PDL):** Introduced in the 1980s, these are effective for treating birthmarks, scars, and vascular conditions such as port-wine stains and rosacea.[59] They typically penetrate around 585 to 595 nm and are specifically absorbed by oxyhemoglobin (the red pigment in blood), allowing the laser to heat and destroy targeted blood vessels without significantly affecting surrounding tissue. This makes it ideal for treating surface-level skin issues without damaging deeper layers. It is a great workhorse of a machine.

When to use laser treatment

There are many scenarios for which lasering is a great option. Focusing on the face specifically, there is an order I typically like to follow. First, I use a BBL to clean up pigment disorders such as melasma or lentigos (age spots), along with telangiectasias (capillaries/blood vessels). This type of laser is also great for light age spots that look like freckles. If a patient has rosacea or acne, I would focus on that too. In addition to correcting pigment, this treatment also begins to tighten up loose collagen, which is where we start to see the benefits of looking more youthful.

If a patient is still having clinical deficits in their skin, including tactile texture, pores, or tightness, I recommend a laser more like Moxi, Halo, or total resurfacing.

In general, you want to use the least-invasive laser that will get the job done. If a patient has never had lasering and we don't know how they will respond, I take a conservative approach to their treatment. Less is more. After the initial treatment, we can adjust from there for any future appointments.

The best strategy for aesthetic treatments in general is to focus on prevention and maintenance rather than correcting more serious issues later. When patients are doing an annual aesthetic update, I almost always recommend including laser treatment. That's because when the skin is tighter, other treatments will work better. A good example of this is Botox. Botox freezes the muscles so the skin doesn't wrinkle as much, but the skin is still getting looser and losing elasticity.

When not to use laser treatment

Laser treatments aren't for everyone. It's incredibly important to safeguard against the risk of complications. People who have Fitzpatrick type I skin are more sensitive, and their treatment should be adjusted appropriately. These are the patients whose skin could swell tremendously and must be advised of this prior to treatment.

Patients with underlying autoimmune diseases can experience complications with lasers as well since their bodies can't heal the micro injuries as well and recover properly. It's important for practitioners to make this abundantly clear to them. (Even if you have this spelled out in the fine print on your release forms, there's no guarantee that your patients will read and understand the risks.) Always have a conversation about this before providing laser treatment and remember to ask returning patients if they have had any changes to their health.

If you fail to properly screen these types of patients and provide a service that is too strong for them to handle, it's possible that their skin could become red and inflamed for a month or more after the treatment. Having this much downtime will come as a very unpleasant and painful surprise.

Lastly, lasering should not be done too soon before or after getting Botox or other injections as it can cause swelling, which affects how the product settles. I like to schedule these services at least a week apart.

Pre- and post-care instructions

Following specific instructions before and after getting treatment can make a major difference in both pain and outcomes. Here are some of the key instructions to share with patients before they come in for their treatment:

- **Avoid sun exposure:** Stay out of direct sunlight for at least two to four weeks before the procedure. If you need to be outdoors, use a broad-spectrum sunscreen with an SPF of 30 or higher.

- **Discontinue certain medications:** Stop using medications that increase photosensitivity (e.g., certain antibiotics and acne medications) at least a week before treatment—but only under the guidance of your healthcare practitioner. Avoid blood-thinning medications (e.g., aspirin and ibuprofen) for at least a week before the procedure to reduce the risk of bruising and bleeding.

- **Skincare products:** Discontinue the use of retinoids, AHAs, and other exfoliating or irritating products a few days before treatment. Use gentle cleansers and moisturizers to keep the skin hydrated.

- **Numbing:** We often let patients know that they have the option of having us apply numbing cream when they arrive to make their treatment more comfortable.

Here are some of the instructions we share with patients on how to take care of themselves after treatment:

- **Cooling and soothing:** Cold compresses or ice packs can be used to reduce swelling and discomfort immediately after the procedure. A spray bottle filled with water is another nice option.
- **Sun protection:** Avoid direct sun exposure for at least two weeks after treatment. Use a broad-spectrum sunscreen with an SPF of 30 or higher and wear protective clothing and hats whenever outdoors. (This is crucial for maintaining results! You can "undo" those months the laser took off your face by spending just an hour or two in the sun right after treatment.) I encourage my patients to use a sunscreen that also blocks blue light and infrared rays.
- **Gentle skincare:** Your skin will be tender, and the products you usually use might burn or cause irritation. Use a gentle cleanser and avoid scrubbing or exfoliating the treated area. Apply a gentle moisturizer regularly to keep the skin hydrated and to aid in healing. My favorite product after lasering to soothe the skin is hyaluronic acid. There are also a number of products available to help boost healing post-lasering. Pick one for your patients and have a system in place. We recently pivoted to using exosomes directly after laser treatments and encouraging patients to continue this at home during this post-operative period.[60]
- **Avoid irritating products:** Avoid using retinoids, AHAs, BHAs, and other active ingredients until your skin has fully healed, typically for one to two weeks. Avoid using makeup for at least 24 hours or until any redness or swelling subsides.
- **No picking or scratching:** Do not pick at or scratch the treated area, as doing so can lead to scarring and infection.
- **Avoid heat:** Avoid hot showers, saunas, and vigorous exercise for at least 24 to 48 hours post-treatment to prevent irritation and swelling.

Investment

I would be remiss if I didn't bring up pricing in this chapter. Laser machines often cost $200,000 or more. This is a hefty up-front cost for aesthetic treatment practitioners and a key reason why more practitioners don't offer any laser services, or only offer one or two types of lasers that they use for all their patients.

Although laser machines are expensive, the cost per use is much lower than other treatments, which means the profitability of providing laser treatments can ultimately be much higher than from other services. The manufacturers I've purchased from have always been very good about providing the financial modeling for various levels of use and pricing so that my team and I have a thorough understanding of our investment and the risk we would be taking on. (Keep in mind that laser machines are built to last for decades, so purchasing one is definitely a long-term investment.)

Also be aware that in addition to buying the laser machine, there are often consumables that are used and will need to be repurchased. Some lasers, such as Moxi and BBL Heroic, now have a crystal head or a needled head that is used for a certain number of pulses. Depending on how often you use the machine, you might need to replace the crystal head more often, maybe even every six weeks or so. The companies that produce these lasers also have insurance policies that they offer for this purpose, and you can do the math to see whether this might be a benefit to your practice. Our practice found this plan to be worth the investment.

Whenever I decide to buy a new laser, I consider whether it will be filling a gap in our current treatments or will enable me to help a certain demographic of patients more than our current machines do. It's also important to point out that some machines offer "two-in-one" or even "three-in-one" functionality and can operate on different wavelengths to serve different purposes.

My office has the Cynosure Vectus hair-removal laser, Sciton BBL Joule with Nd:YAG and erbium laser, Sciton BBL Heroic with Moxi, Forever Bare, SkinTyte, Forever Young, and the Candela PDL. This combination allows us to make the right recommendation for each patient, rather than using machines that are either too strong or not strong enough to achieve the ideal results. If you're only going to buy one laser, I recommend the BBL Heroic with Moxi, or something that serves a similar purpose.

Light therapy

Blue-light therapy

Blue light operates to around 400–500 nm and targets the skin's surface. It's effective in killing bacteria, which helps treat acne, oily skin, and clogged pores. For those with chronic blemishes, blue-light therapy can be an easy way to get clearer skin naturally.

Red-light therapy

Red light operates to around 630–700 nm, which penetrates deeper into the skin than blue light does. Red-light therapy is primarily used for anti-aging and healing. It helps increase collagen production, reduces inflammation and redness (e.g., rosacea), and improves skin texture. It can treat fine lines and wrinkles in a gentler way than lasers can.

Another major benefit of red-light therapy is treatments for hair growth. Both men and women of all ages can experience hair loss, and it's a stressful thing for people to have to go through. I've spoken with hair-loss experts who say treatments are not what they used to be, but it is still possible to regrow your hair.

Red-light therapy works by penetrating the scalp and improving circulation around hair follicles, delivering more oxygen and nutrients that are essential for hair growth. This increased blood flow helps nourish and revitalize dormant or weakened hair follicles. It also stimulates cellular activity, which helps hair follicles shift from the resting phase (telogen) back to the growth phase (anagen), encouraging new hair growth. Additionally, if a person is actively losing their hair, red-light therapy can prevent the hair follicles from scarring over.

There are many different companies that offer light technology—for both professionals and at-home use. Professional machines allow practitioners to adjust the settings and provide customized treatment for patients. They also tend to be much more effective than at-home devices.

To treat most conditions, consistent use is typically necessary to see noticeable results. That said, patients should not overdo it. Frequent, ongoing exposure to light can damage the skin. I know someone who has a $20,000 at-home red-light-therapy machine and her skin looks much older than her age. When it comes to any area of aesthetics, more is not always more.

A look at the future

Light and laser-therapy services are treatment options that haven't gotten the attention they deserve. This area of aesthetics is still widely misunderstood and/or overlooked by many patients. It's a shame, because advances in technology have made these treatments not only highly effective but also accessible for a wide range of skin concerns—from acne to wrinkles to hair regrowth and scar reduction. Light and laser therapies offer non-invasive, science-backed solutions that can deliver impressive results.

If, as a practitioner, you haven't leaned into lasers and light therapy, I encourage you to do so. The machines can be a bit of an investment, but they do pay off in the long term and provide the outcomes that a large percentage of patients want.

CHAPTER 8

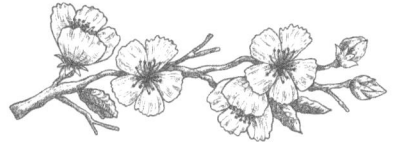

Botox

I was in dermatology residency at the University of Iowa in 2003 when my professor told the residents that we would be getting special training by a man named Dr. Alastair Carruthers. He and his wife, Dr. Jean Carruthers, were doing amazing work with a new neuromodulator called botulinum toxin, and it was sure to change the industry as we knew it.

Doctors and researchers had been studying botulinum toxin for many years and were finding numerous medical uses for it. In one case, it was used to treat eye spasms. A patient in 1987 noticed that when she was treated, she developed a "beautiful, untroubled expression."[61] In other words, her wrinkles faded away.

Upon hearing this, the Carrutherses became interested in whether botulinum toxin could be used purely for cosmetic purposes. Jean noticed that their receptionist had a deep line between her eyebrows that looked to her like "a crevasse by about two in the afternoon." Jean asked her if she could try injecting her in that area. The receptionist agreed. Three days later, they were all amazed at the results.[62]

Jean and Alastair wanted to spread the word and get more patients, but people were understandably reluctant to get a substance that was essentially poison injected into their face. It took many years of research and hard work, but 16 years later, Botox was finally approved for cosmetic use. Understanding the potential of the product, my residency program wanted to train students on how it works and where to inject it.

Flash forward a couple decades and I'm still honored to have been trained by one of the godfathers of Botox. As this book was being written, we learned of his passing and particularly wanted to thank his wife and family for all of his pioneering contributions to this aesthetics space. Today, Botox is easily the most popular aesthetic treatment worldwide. With more than 5,200 studies conducted, it is also the most studied neuromodulator in the world. It has earned a devoted following from an incredibly wide demographic of people. The relatively low cost, speed of treatment, widespread availability, and noticeable results in terms of decreasing dynamic lines and wrinkles have made it a gateway treatment for patients to enter the aesthetics space.

The science

Botulinum toxin type A is a neurotoxin that is produced by the bacterium *Clostridium botulinum* and has the following properties:

- **Neurotoxin effect:** It works by blocking the release of acetylcholine, a neurotransmitter responsible for muscle contraction. When injected into specific muscles, botulinum toxin type A prevents them from contracting, leading to a temporary reduction in muscle activity.
- **Wrinkle reduction:** By paralyzing the underlying muscles, botulinum toxin type A smooths out the skin above, reducing the appearance of dynamic wrinkles and fine lines caused by repetitive facial movements. (Botox is not used for static lines.)

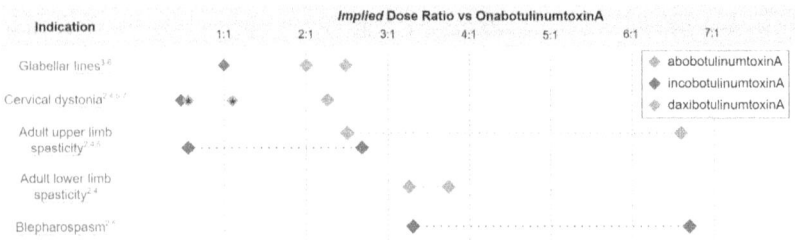

The product behaves very differently depending on the area of the body where the different types of botulinum toxin type A is injected.

Brands

Like Kleenex and Band-Aid, Botox is a brand name that people often use to describe similar products. Many people outside the aesthetics industry don't realize that there are actually numerous types of botulinum toxin type A, including Botox, Dysport, Xeomin, Jeuveau, and Daxxify.

These products are all studied individually. Although they do work in similar ways, many practitioners aren't aware that they are not exact substitutes, as the molecules of each behave differently in various parts of the body. Some products spread out more than others do, which creates varying effects. In other words, if you're used to injecting Dysport in patients and you switch to Jeuveau, your results are likely to look different even if you inject in exactly the same way. Another reason this happens is because the potency of the products isn't standardized, which means the units aren't identical. If you inject 64 units of Botox into a patient and then switch to 64 units of Xeomin, you aren't injecting exactly the same potency of botulinum toxin type A, which is likely to yield different results.

For these reasons, I highly recommend that all aesthetic practitioners who provide botulinum toxin type A pick a single brand and stick to it so they can become masters in their craft with that one product. That's what I've done with Botox. By choosing a single product, I've been able to eliminate unnecessary variables and hone my craft with a high level of precision.

And just to be crystal clear, since Botox is a specific product rather than a type of treatment, if you choose to provide another brand, you cannot legally market it as "Botox," which would be false advertising and misrepresentation.

In this book, when I talk about "Botox," I am indeed referring to the brand Botox rather than other brands of botulinum toxin type A. That said, whatever brand you choose to work with, the advice in this chapter will be helpful for you.

Overall, there has been an exponential demand for Botox in recent years. It's become a household name and earned a reputation for being safe and reliable. Though many patients are closed-lipped about the types of aesthetic services they receive, a growing number are fully transparent that they regularly get Botox. Any stigma around it is quickly disappearing, and it's turning into a mainstream beauty-maintenance service, much like going to the hairdresser.

The effect this has had on the industry has been interesting, to say the least! It's important for practitioners and patients to understand the trends and what it means for them.

When there's a growing consumer demand for a product or service, there's also a huge opportunity for practitioners to enter the market and expand their business. We've seen this at scale. It seems like everyone provides Botox these days. It originated in dermatology and plastic-surgery offices, and now it's in med spas and used by dentists and a host of other medical specialists. And it's easy to see why! Becoming decent at injecting Botox isn't particularly difficult, and it's a quick service to provide. Botox is an excellent way for aesthetic practitioners to connect with patients who are brand new to the space—and to secure repeat business. It's also an easy upsell for practitioners who are already providing other services to patients.

All these reasons show why so much lobbying has been done across the country to make state laws less restrictive when it comes to the requirements needed for administering botulinum toxin type A. It's safe, patients want it, and more practitioners are needed to meet the growing demand. Nationwide, we've seen lawmakers respond to this situation by pulling back restrictions to allow practitioners with different types of licensing to provide botulinum toxin type A.

This has shifted the landscape. Botulinum toxin type A is now widely available, and the number of injections per year only keeps increasing. For practitioners, this means there are more customers—and also more competition.

As more and more people administer Botox, it's becoming a commodity. Simply offering Botox isn't enough to differentiate yourself and alone won't keep your business afloat in the long term.

Many practitioners try to compete by offering lower pricing. This can be an OK strategy if you think of Botox as a loss leader for your business. It's like the rotisserie chickens at Costco. The margins would be too low for the business to survive if they only sold rotisserie chickens, but customers also buy the membership and a cart full of other groceries. And even better, some buy numerous bottles of wine, which are strategically placed near the chicken and have a much higher markup.[63]

At my dermatology office, Botox is only a small portion of our business. We choose to keep prices low because it's an important part of our mix of services. Many new patients come in through our doors because they are interested in Botox. Once my team and I meet with them, we determine whether they are, in fact, great candidates for Botox and it's the best treatment to yield the desired results. As we learn more about their needs and concerns, it often makes sense for many patients to try other services as well, whether in the short or long term. For example, everyone older than 40 (as well as younger patients who are high risk) should be getting an annual full-body skin check. Safety is my top priority, so I always use the opportunity to help make sure Botox patients are taking care of their annual wellness appointments. From there, since these patients are interested in having a more youthful appearance, many are curious to learn about alternative aesthetic services that could complement their Botox, such as other fillers or lasering services. I find that a combination of a couple modalities often drives the results that really wow patients. This approach enables us to offer Botox at competitive prices while growing a profitable practice.

If you try to compete based on price with Botox and it's a significant percentage of your business, you'll be on a slippery slope as you'll be competing with other practitioners who are positioning Botox as a loss leader, which means your margins will be incredibly low with little else to make up for it.

When this happens, practitioners are tempted to source products for a lower cost. There are a variety of ways to do this. When you buy a higher quantity of vials of Botox, the price per unit goes down. This is the smartest way to go, but even then, the prices won't be that much lower.

Wholesale Botox is pretty price stable, meaning the cost doesn't fluctuate much and it won't go on sale. This is reflected in how authorized retailers price Botox. However, if you search online, you'll likely find all kinds of deals through websites you've never heard of, both in the United States and abroad.

As a practitioner, whenever you buy Botox (or any other brand of botulinum toxin type A), you must buy it from an authorized seller. Even if a website looks legitimate and you've heard of other practitioners using it to get better pricing, don't assume it's the real product or that it's safe to use. If it seems too good to be true, it probably is.

When you're injecting something under the skin, it's vital to ensure that you're using the right product. Counterfeit Botox has penetrated the market, and it's risky and scary for everyone involved. Patients have become disfigured and died from it, and practitioners have lost their licenses and even gone to jail.

One infamous case happened here in South Dakota, wherein the dermatologist lost his license for five years. His staff member who was in charge of purchasing bought a Botox-like product from an unapproved seller. She only bought six vials. Unfortunately, the drug was a different form of botulinum A that was only approved for research by the FDA, rather than being approved for use with patients. The government found out and sent his office a query letter. Due to poor office management and carelessness, the letter fell through the cracks and he failed to respond to the FDA within the prescribed timeframe. He was debarred for five years, which is a horror story that should serve as a warning to all of us.

Authentic Botox vials always come with a specific hologram on them to denote their authenticity. Familiarize yourself with what this looks like, and make sure you always check every bottle.

You might be able to find other brands of botulinum toxin type A for a lower price than Botox or take advantage of sales from authorized sellers, but as mentioned earlier, it isn't recommended to switch back and forth between different brands because the products aren't apples to apples and you won't get the same results. Further, it is dishonest and illegal to market a service as "Botox" for the brand recognition and then inject a different product.

Patients should feel empowered to ask practitioners to see their botulinum toxin type A vials at the time of treatment to ensure that they're getting what they expect. This should not be seen as an annoyance by practitioners. If everyone becomes more conscious of safety, there will only be better outcomes.

Become a master injector

There's so much more to Botox than most people realize. Yes, it does wonders for forehead wrinkles, but that's only the tip of the iceberg. The recommendations on where and how to use Botox have changed considerably, especially in recent years. Guidelines used to be quite limited, but they've expanded in unexpected ways. Today, patients are getting better outcomes than ever before, and I expect this trend to continue as new research comes out and practitioners keep honing their craft. This is important news for all of us.

As practitioners, we need to keep seeking new information and training to help us provide the best possible outcomes for our patients. And from a business standpoint, becoming an expert has always been a successful way to stand out from the competition in a crowded space. Not only will this bring more patients in the door and keep them coming back, but it also reduces the need to compete based on price.

If you charge more than your competitors do but your expertise and the patient experience you provide set you apart, Botox will no longer be seen as a commodity to your patients. Your patients will understand that they aren't just paying for the product—they're paying for the expertise of the person administering it.

As more and more patients become educated on the advanced techniques available for Botox, the demand for master injectors will continue to rise. And practitioners who have top-notch skills will have a clear advantage.

A new approach

The most common (and original) places to cosmetically inject Botox are all within the top-third section of the face. We've been targeting forehead lines, frown lines, and crow's feet for decades. But what about the bottom two-thirds? No one wants to look 10 years older from the nose down! Thankfully, new strategies and recommendations for injections develop over time as practitioners try their hand at different techniques, after which the formal research follows.

It's important to note that there are hundreds of opinions out there regarding how much Botox people need on average and where to place it—and there is no single right answer because everyone's face and body are different.

To start, it's important to make sure your patient is a good fit for Botox; the best candidates will have good skin quality. The on-label recommendation is that Botox should only be used for people who are under 65. When patients have too much rough or sagging skin (especially in the jowls), Botox alone will not produce the outcomes they want.

For patients who would be good Botox candidates in the future if their skin quality were to improve, I often recommend doing a laser treatment, or a series of laser treatments, first. After the skin becomes tighter is when we move on to Botox. It's important that I thoroughly explain this to patients so they understand I'm not trying to upsell them. I tell them directly that I do not want them to be disappointed by their treatment, which is what is likely to happen if we were to start with Botox.

At my practice, we frequently follow the "rule of three" for routine Botox patients, injecting 64 units across the face in three areas: 20 in the forehead, 20 in crow's feet, and 12 around each eye. Through many years of experience, as well as from research and recommendations from the industry, we've found this to be the ideal treatment for the majority of our patients. To maintain results, we recommend having it done three times per year.

For new patients, as well as patients who want to achieve specific outcomes outside general aging maintenance, I often come up with a custom plan to target different areas, injecting Botox in all kinds of places that people find surprising, including the upper lip, chin, jawline, and neck. Some of these areas require a great deal of finesse and expertise to do well.

A breakdown of some of my best strategies

In the following section, I've included some great tips and tricks for injecting Botox in general, as well as techniques specifically for various areas of the face.

Hyperdilution: I make a thinner product by mixing more saline into the Botox, and then I inject it very superficially under the skin in tiny amounts. I've used this approach to successfully address a variety of concerns, including chicken skin on the neck, vertical accordion lines on the cheeks, and rosacea. I usually do a dilution of 4:1 for this area and place one to two units across the accordion lines superficially. I also use this dilution for acne and rosacea of the mid cheeks. You want to see a small blister just under the epidermis for this method. This is a particularly wonderful tool for patients who can't tolerate creams and other medications for acne and rosacea. For example, I have a medical assistant who has severe migraines and can't tolerate oral antibiotics for her rosacea. Her skin is super sensitive, and she has dermatographic urticaria, which means her skin welts easily from being stroked or rubbed. I like to think of these people as my potentially evolving autoimmune folks, so I am super careful about further aggravating their skin with treatments, fragrances, and/or creams. For this particular patient, the rosacea Botox treatment has been a lifesaver.

The lower third of the face: In general, my focus is always rooted in vertical restoration. Dr. Mauricio de Maio, a master injector and someone I've come to respect deeply for his approach to fillers, likes to think of the face as a house, with the cheeks/midface as the foundation and chin and jawline the elevation, with the area around the mouth the final finishing touches. When a patient is bothered by a certain area on their face, the best strategy can often be to treat a different area. I learned a host of lower-face applications from his techniques and would highly recommend any of his training courses.

Chin: Look into the mirror, roll your bottom lip out and under, and make "that face." In my clinic, we call it "baby cry." I have a wonderful nurse who volunteered to make this face and many others for photos we keep on hand at the clinic. We have these images lined up on a laminated card that we ask our patients to hold while they mimic the faces to help us determine where Botox could be of benefit. Find me a woman who likes how her chin looks while making this face and I will be amazed. It's not flattering. One of the reasons this mentalis (lower lip) muscle gets bigger as we age is that our bone under this area gets resorbed. The muscle compensates to allow function of the orbicularis oris muscle (another muscle that controls the lips); it's the scaffolding support. We treat this *peau d'orange* tissue (had to use this wording to make my minor in French relevant!) with Botox to diminish the appearance of orange-peel skin on the chin (dimpling) and return to a more youthful look. However, this often also needs to be addressed with underlying filler replacement. (See the chapter on filler for more information on the technique.)

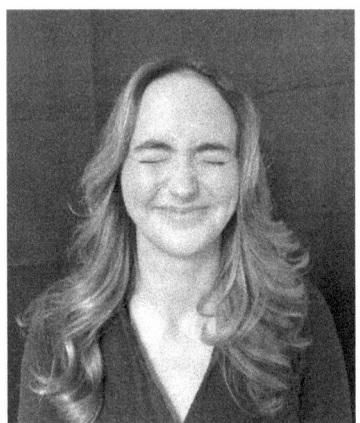

Squint

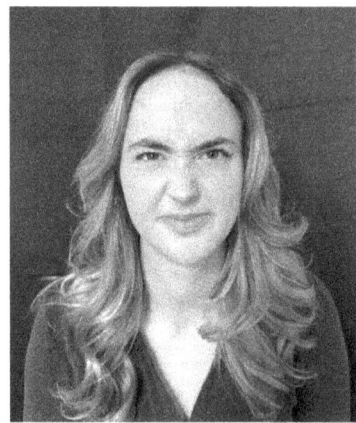

Bunny Lines

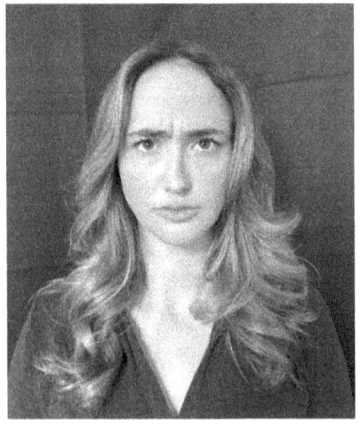

Scowl

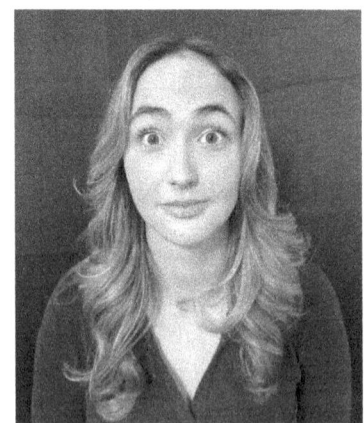

Surprised

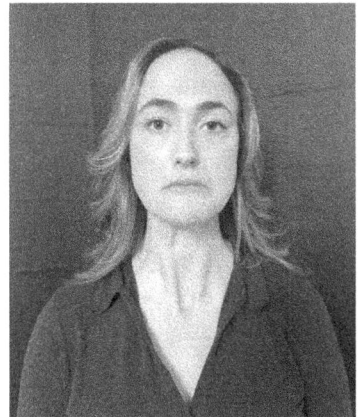
Platysmal Bands

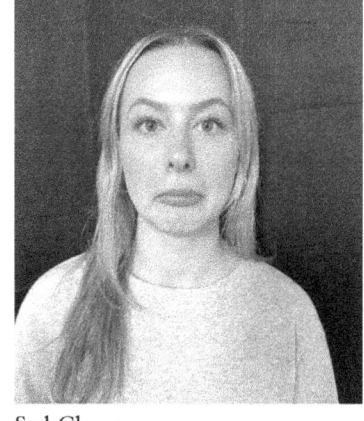
Sad Clown

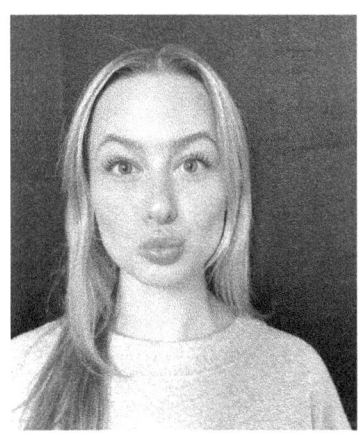
Kissy Face

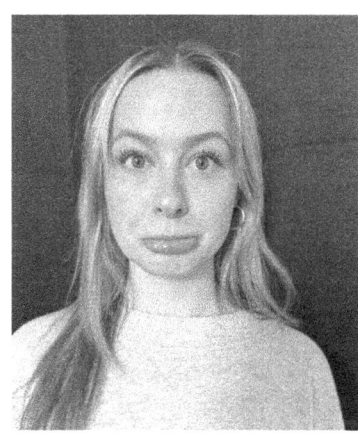
Baby Cry

    The mentalis muscle can be tricky because it is next to the depressor labii inferioris (DLI) muscle, and if we accidently hit it, the patient's smile will be lopsided on animation (movement). This risk is often a deterrent for those who administer Botox, and many people just don't want to inject there. Creating a lopsided smile is certainly a risk, but there are simple steps to avoid it. First off, using the right technique to aim at the center of the mentalis makes it very unlikely you'll get asymmetrical results. But if that does happen, I've found that using a hot pack along with vigorous massage a couple times a day to the affected area for a few days will usually reverse the majority of the issue.

Lateral to the DLI is the depressor anguli oris (DAO), which *is* a muscle we want to address if a patient has a prominent pulling down of the lateral corners of their mouth when frowning. I usually use a 1:1 dilution when working on the lower third of the face. I also use one to two units on each side for younger patients and up to four units per side for my more mature patients. It's a game changer that can even reduce the appearance of jowls.

Jawline: Treating the jawline can be important, especially when that part of the face is pulling down the top third of the face. Remember, everything in the body is connected. When we treat one area, it can affect another. Treating the jawline can release tension in that area and the upper neck, which reduces the pull on the top third of the face. (I've seen how this can often eliminate or greatly reduce the need for injecting filler into the cheeks.)

In addition to using Botox for help with vertical restoration, one thing that ages people considerably is the appearance of jowls. That's the extra saggy skin than hangs from the jawline into the neck. In my practice, I have been using Botox in the jawline to add definition and reduce the appearance of jowls, which does wonders for creating a more youthful appearance.

A great deal of research was performed on treating the jawline with Botox between 2008 and 2017. I've read a couple dozen papers from around the world, and my favorite procedure is the Nefertiti lift.

Despite the significant research on using Botox in the jawline, it's still not a strategy that has been widely used off-label. However, with FDA approval for this area pending, we can expect this to be an area of growth when it comes to Botox. I believe that the final protocol coming out from Allergan will be a reflection of the best learnings from the international literature.

Masseters: Many of my patients who clench their teeth often also have more lines around their mouth and develop a "pinched-up look" at times. They can even clench so hard that they create craze lines or damage their teeth. These patients are close to my heart as I also have this problem. For me, it became apparent when my mom was passing away and in hospice and I suffered from horrible headaches and started cracking my teeth. I could not do much about my stress as I was working full time in South Dakota, had three kids at home, and was traveling back and forth to City of Hope in California almost every weekend to be with my mom. It was a grueling trek, and it took a toll.

It was also a wake-up call for me to learn more about how to protect myself from stress, learn to meditate, and, of course, prevent future cracks in my teeth. After a deep dive into the dental literature, I discovered that injecting my masseter (jaw) muscles would be very helpful and a watershed for headaches.

I now inject my patients in the same way. I start by doing two to three injections of 15 to 20 units on each masseter. Some patients also need injections to the temporalis muscle.[64] Ask them to chew for you, and if they have visible bulging, they are your candidates for one to two additional units on each side of that muscle.

Around the eyes: Many of us have been injecting our periorbital area for a while. However, I would say that my technique has greatly evolved over the last 18 to 24 months. This is an area in which I am really having fun with the evolution of my practice. I have stopped going as deep as I used to go and instead have been focusing more on superficial injections. This is especially true for my patients who are bothered by the appearance of their hooded eyes. I often inject Botox under the eyebrows, about one third of the way in from the tail of each one. When patients want their eyes to appear more open, I do a trick of 1:1 dilution with one unit to the mid infra eyelid margin and one to the lateral eyelid margin. These shots go way up there—close to the actual margin—and are transformational.

For people who feel like their glabella (the area between their eyebrows) is persistent despite FDA proper dosing, I have been targeting deeper centrally and sometimes on the medial orbicularis oculi.

It's important to note that the eyes are the riskiest area of the body when it comes to fillers in general; however, Botox doesn't pose the same level of risk because it won't cause blindness. The molecule for Botox is smaller, and it works in a different way than other fillers, but you still have to be careful injecting it. If muscles around the eyelid are affected, it can cause ptosis, where the eyelids droop. This can affect the aesthetic outcome as well as a patient's vision. Given the relatively short lifespan of Botox, results are not permanent, but practitioners should still use caution.

Forehead: The forehead muscles have been a key target for Botox from the beginning, and the procedure is often considered to be fairly straightforward and low risk. That said, all the muscles in the face are connected. Freezing muscles in one area, especially on a long-term basis, can cause unintended effects.

A common pitfall has been if you inject too low (below the line of convergence), it can cause the eyebrows and eyelids to droop. Also, I have noticed that some patients who are underdosed persistently in this area (especially those who have a wider frontalis muscle) can develop new wrinkles. That's because when you continue injecting too close to the midline, the muscles near the sides of the face can end up working harder than they otherwise would, which can create a rainbow wrinkle effect. To safeguard against this, move injections farther to the outside of the face so that the muscles in that area are also frozen. Filler can also be used in the temples to support this area and achieve better results.

Neck: In addition to smoothing the skin through hyperdilution, Botox can be used to improve the appearance of platysma bands in the neck. This strategy is hot off the presses from Allergan, which means you can now receive training from them directly on how to leverage it. I often use this technique with the jawline definition as well.

Lip flip: To add volume in the top lip and give the appearance of a ski jump, I inject Botox into the very top of the upper lip. This lip-flip strategy is usually recommended for women in their mid 30s and younger. For women who are older than this, I tend to pivot and go a little higher and inject midway up on the cutaneous lip. This addresses the lines that can be perceived as "smoker's lines."

Smile support: When patients are concerned that they have a "gummy smile" that shows too much teeth and gums, I inject high on their upper lip, actually almost to the top of the melolabial skin fold, to drop the lip when they smile. Other patients say that their smile looks more like a sneer, and I treat that unilaterally by injecting just lateral to the nose. For horizontal lines on the upper cutaneous lip, I stay medial but just under the introitus (opening) to the nostril.

Lines around the sides of the mouth: Patients are often bothered by what we refer to as "sad-clown lines." This is one of the most common places to get dynamic wrinkles as we age. I mentioned this in the section about the chin, because it so often goes along with the chin, but sometimes patients might just need their DAOs treated. You can test this by asking the patient to make that sad-clown face. If it's really prominent but they don't have any "orange peel" on their chin, they don't need their chin treated and just need their DAOs treated.

Bunny lines on the nose: Lots of us talk about the bunny lines these days. When I first started injecting Botox as a treatment for them, I was trained to target the nasalis muscle, which is really only responsible for sniffing. A better technique is to target the LLSAN muscle (levator labii superioris alaeque nasalis) muscle around the eyes.

I think the most famous person I noticed 15 or so years ago who didn't appear to treat her bunny lines was Meg Ryan. Her smile looked like her frown. She couldn't emote properly. I think treating her bunny lines would have fixed that. It highlights that even movie stars might not have access to the latest techniques. She also made news recently over plastic surgery that she had done as well. It must be difficult to be in the public eye constantly!

Symmetry: It's important to inject symmetrically so that the patient doesn't develop results that are inconsistent on each side of the face. That said, most faces aren't symmetrical. For the most part, I don't tend to chase symmetry where it doesn't naturally exist. However, when you're doing complex injections and working with a significantly asymmetrical palette, you will need to adjust your approach. It's possible that one side of the face might need a little more Botox than the other. This can happen when people sleep on one side, animate with a "sneer," or perhaps spend a lot of time driving and have the sun on the left side of their face.

Moderation: As companies have devoted many resources working through dose, duration studies, and FDA approvals, I tend to follow the recommendations that so many scientists have worked hard to formulate. One reason I find this important is that botulinum toxin type A isn't recommended for frequent, continued dosing. Although rare, using this product more than three times per year can increase the likelihood that someone becomes immune to it. Injectors are often at the biggest risk of this because many of us microdose regularly! Note that the recommendation here is not brand specific; it's three times per year total, not three times per year per brand.

How to make Botox last longer

It's important that you make sure your patients know how to get the most out of their treatments, including the following:

- Take your zinc. As noted in chapter 4, taking zinc every day is an easy way to get more mileage out of your Botox.
- Cut back on stress. The more stressful a time period has been for me, the more I am animating (moving) my face. It's not always noticeable when this is happening in my day-to-day, but the long-term effect is that my Botox wears off more quickly. I have heard this for many years from my patients as well.

Fast-acting Botox—NEW!

There's a new type of botulinum toxin entering the market from Allergan. Botulinum toxin type E works quicker, provides results within hours, and lasts a month. This is a great option for people who want a little pick-me-up right before an important event. It's also a powerful tool for patients to experiment with in new areas to see if it's a match for their aesthetic before they commit to traditional Botox. I can also imagine that it will be available at a lower price point and that patients will be able to see what an outcome might look like for them with full FDA-approved dosing.

Note that patients who have immunity to botulinum toxin A won't automatically have immunity to type E. At a recent cosmetic meeting in Beverly Hills, several of the other injectors at the breakout sessions noted how excited they were to give their systems a break and try the new Botox E.

Even though I've been injecting Botox for more than 20 years, I'm still curious to learn more about this new type E! I actively pursue advanced training opportunities through meetings, including AAD, the American Society of Dermatologic Surgery, other cosmetic meetings, and online webinars. I especially enjoy the trainings from Allergan. A recent treat was the one they recently aired with Dr. Jean Carruthers. I also stay involved in the aesthetics community to keep abreast of new research and follow some of the top Botox injectors in the world, such as Murad Alam, MD; Saami Khalifian, MD; Mauricio de Maio, MD; Jeanine Downie, MD; Leslie Fletcher, NP; Sabrina Fabi, MD; Julie Bass Kaplan, CNP; Katie O'Brien, PA-C; and Nicola Lowrey, PA-C, at meetings and on social media. By taking educational courses, following a variety of injectors on social media for tips, and attending aesthetic dermatology conferences, I'm always learning and trying new techniques that help me keep leveling up my expertise to benefit my patients. If you inject Botox, I implore you to do the same!

Think of Botox as an art. Anyone can hold a paintbrush and put color on a canvas, but it takes an incredible amount of practice and skill to execute certain techniques and create a masterpiece. And that's what we should all be striving for, right? Not just smoothing foreheads and getting patients in and out the door quickly. We should be going above and beyond to see how Botox, a key tool in our tool kit, can create results that exceed expectations.

Chapter 9

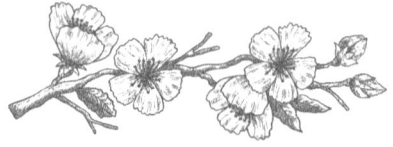

Filler

Gladys Deacon was the "it" girl of the early 1900s. The belle of many balls, she was known for her big blue eyes and rare beauty. Leaders at the Pond's beauty-cream company saw that she was special when they hired her to be the face of their products as a model. There was just something about her that captivated attention.

Gladys had a "celebrity" crush from the time she was a teenager: the Duke of Marlborough. Though she was courted by numerous men of high society, she had her sights set on the duke. Sure enough, she had the beauty and confidence to pursue him, and she ended up marrying him to become the Dutchess of Marlborough.

Gladys had it all, but as she entered her 20s, she was concerned that her looks were fading. She heard about a revolutionary beauty treatment wherein paraffin wax was being injected under the skin to enhance features. She wanted to try it to get rid of the "kink" she'd complained about in her nose and achieve a perfect "Grecian profile." So at the ripe age of 22, she traveled to Paris and got the injections. Much to her horror, the wax ended up falling into her chin and settling there, creating a bumpy, misshapen appearance.

This would be traumatizing for anyone, but for Gladys, it marked the beginning of her life as a recluse. She retreated from her husband, family, and society. She took to keeping a loaded gun by her bed and threatened to shoot her husband if he did so much as come in her room to look at her. He left her alone in the palace for two years before finally evicting her. Ultimately, she moved into an isolated farmhouse and then a psychiatric hospital, where she died in 1977 at 96 years old.[65]

We think of filler as being a relatively new aesthetic treatment, but it's actually been around since the late 1800s, shortly after the invention of the syringe.[66] First, people were injecting paraffin and Vaseline; then they moved on to silicone, then bovine collagen, and then the many options we have today. It took us a little time to get here, but the products and technology *The ability to mold and shape the face while maintaining harmony with natural features and contours requires both technical skill and a keen eye for aesthetics.* have come a long way, especially as it relates to safety, reliability of results, and protocols for addressing adverse outcomes. Although there have certainly been bumps along the way (no pun intended), filler has become one of the most popular aesthetic treatments. Whether it's adding volume to the lips, contouring the cheeks, or smoothing out fine lines and wrinkles, filler provides subtle yet meaningful enhancements that patients love.

Injecting filler truly is an art form! The ability to mold and shape the face while maintaining harmony with natural features and contours requires both technical skill and a keen eye for aesthetics. Each patient has unique facial anatomy, meaning that no two procedures are exactly the same. This is where the nuance of filler comes into play: practitioners need to not only understand the anatomy but also have a sense of balance, proportion, and symmetry to create natural-looking results that enhance a patient's features rather than overwhelm or detract from them.

For new practitioners, this can be intimidating. The sheer customization involved in filler treatments means there's much room for error if the technique isn't spot-on. Misplacing filler by even a few millimeters or failing to understand how the filler is likely to migrate can create unintended results that dramatically alter a person's appearance. Or worse, injecting filler can create a vascular occlusion.

The most important thing to understand is that education and training make a huge difference in results. It takes time, experience, and constant learning to develop the knowledge and precision needed to achieve consistent, beautiful results. The learning curve may feel steep, but with patience and dedication, practitioners can transform their technical skills into true artistry, delivering results that exceed patients' expectations.

How to inject

Make sure you have a good conversation with your patients about the features they want to enhance. Push them for specifics in what they are looking for so that you don't make any incorrect assumptions. From there, here are a few key things to keep in mind:

Pick the right brands: Some practitioners inject a variety of brands and types of filler. This can be appealing for patients who come in asking for a certain type of filler by name because they've heard good things about it or had positive results from past treatments. Working with a variety of fillers can also give practitioners more tools in their toolbox when it comes to helping patients. That said, it takes a lot of time to develop a deep understanding of the nuances of how each product works and to truly master it. Some practitioners have the interest and skill to go this direction, but it's important to know that this isn't the only option!

    I wanted to become an expert at injecting a single line of products rather than bouncing around to different options. Instead of having more tools in the toolbox, I chose to focus on mastering fewer tools. After doing a lot of research, I decided to use Allergan's products. Renowned Brazilian plastic surgeon Dr. Maurico de Maio has also done the same with his practice, as have many others. A deciding factor for me was when I read a paper showing that the Juvéderm collection of fillers integrates with the skin, whereas competitors' product just sits on the bone.[67] After that, I switched to using Allergan products only. Although I'm sticking to one brand, I'm still able to use a variety of fillers that are designed to yield nuanced outcomes, and I don't feel as though I need any other tools to create the best possible results for my patients.

Choose your technique: There are two different schools of thought when it comes to injecting: cannula and needle on bone. There are plenty of talented injectors who are proponents of either side. Personally, I've practiced both methods. I recently went to an in-person training with master injectors Nicola Lowrey, PA-C, and Katie Bader, PA-C, and I learned a lot about the cannula method. Lowrey has pioneered her technique of using an ultrasound to assist in the cannula method, and she is publishing papers on it. I expect quite a bit more innovation to happen in this area in coming years. That being said, there is also a lot of variation. For example, the current on-label training for the temples from Allergan is needle on bone.

I believe in always aspirating before doing any injections on the bone. This helps reduce the risks of vascular occlusions. The technique is to put the needle on the bone, aspirate, and check for a flash of red. If you see red, you've hit a blood vessel or artery. Pull out immediately, apply pressure, ice it, and consult your vascular-occlusion protocol (more on this at the end of the chapter). You might use this technique hundreds of times without ever seeing red. If so, that's great! Keep using this method for safety purposes even if it seems superfluous.

Keep it clean: Filler is a class 3 FDA implantable device. It is medicine. It shouldn't be offered at house parties or next to anyone's pool. When you're injecting filler, you need to be diligent about the cleanliness of the environment, not to mention your own hands and work surface (i.e., the patient's body). As Dr. de Maio would say, "Keep it neurotically clean." Any injections should be done with aseptic technique, being mindful of placement of your hands on hair or any non-cleaned areas.[68]

Patients should always thoroughly wash their face before injections. At my office, we give them a headband, which helps to keep their hair out of their face, and then we instruct them to do a couple passes of washing with a gentle cleanser. Then before we inject, two passes of Puracyn are applied, which is sodium hypochlorous acid. People often tell me that their previous filler practitioner just used alcohol wipes instead of making them wash their face. This is dangerous. Alcohol takes over 30 seconds to kill the germs, and many people don't wait that long before starting to inject. On top of that, you don't want a particle of makeup to accidentally get injected onto the bone, which could create a granuloma.[69] Have them wash their face, and then use an antiseptic technique.

Consider numbing: Filler injections can be painful for patients—but not necessarily so painful that you need to numb. This leaves many practitioners and patients wondering what's best. Personally, I numb patients whenever they are getting injections in their lips or when they are doing Skinvive (more on that ahead) simply because it's so many pokes. I also numb wherever I'm going to do a cannula insertion. I want patients to be able to feel at least a small amount of pain so that if I inject filler onto the bone, it will hurt the patient, thus letting me know I've hit a vessel. It's never ideal for a patient to experience pain during any treatment, but in this case, the pluses outweigh the minuses.

Where to inject

In my training, I have learned that vertical restoration is of the utmost importance. I usually start with the temples, then the midface, and then the jawline. I've broken down specific instructions for strategy and placement in the following sections.

Temples

Many of us have been doing temples for quite some time—especially since MD codes and the release of Juvéderm Voluma XC in 2013, on-label for the midface. Thankfully, this year, it became on-label for temples, which means there will be even more training opportunities for practitioners to get the most benefit out of this product.

Very few people come into my clinic asking for filler in their temples, but it's often exactly what they need in order to address their concerns. Once we fill this area, people comment that their entire face appears lifted. In addition to reducing the hollowing in the temples, it can sharpen the jawline and treat jowls. This overall effect can be quite gratifying for patients.

The kicker here is that you need to adequately fill the temple hollow, which is the area within the ligaments: the superior temporal septum and the inferior temporal septum. Bear with me here because it gets a bit technical. The inferior ligament runs from the root of the helix to the superior lateral orbital rim. The temporal crest runs vertical above this and is a transition of the forehead to the temple. The superior temporal septum runs along the temporal crest. The injection technique that I commonly use is one centimeter up from the orbital rim along the temporal crest and one centimeter posteriorly from the temporal fusion line.

Filling this hollow is held in place by these two septa, and it is important to understand the underlying anatomy and vessels present. There are areas of caution as three branches of the external carotid artery have vascular supply in the temples, and post-injection vascular events are definitely a concern. (See the section on vascular occlusions.)

To find the right injection site in the temples, you typically want to target one centimeter up and one centimeter over from the orbital rim, as outlined above. Finding this spot can seem tricky, especially if you're new to injecting here, so I highly recommend watching training videos and shadowing other practitioners.

The average amount injected into patients in the FDA approval studies was about two syringes per temple. I have found in my practice that for people who suffer from headaches, it works well to separate this out into two sessions. This can ease them into the process as the pressure on the bone can trigger a headache. The other option I do is to cut the Voluma with sterile saline for the temples. I learned this from Nicola Lowery, and the results seem lighter and "fluffier." With this method, I don't have patients complaining of headaches. For patients without a history of migraines and/or headaches, I try to supplement two cubic centimeters per temple from the onset.

Midface

I think the midface, especially right in the apple of the cheek, is the golden spot for injection, and doing so is a pillar in my practice. It helps correct the under-eye hallows, gives lift to the jawline, and makes a huge impact in the overall appearance of the patient's face.

In 2020, Dr. de Maio worked with Allergan to divide the face into scientific code sections that could be referenced for training purposes. This was a paradigm shift! I attended Dr. de Maio's virtual training series that shared the new codes and his strategies for injecting the midface, and it blew me away. Filler is a real workhorse when you use it this way. It gives structure to the midface and can look just like a facelift.

After I started implementing his strategies, I could tell that I was leveling up my skill a ton. In fact, my longtime representative who is now a part of Allergan Medical Institute told me, "2020 was a HUGE growth year for you. I knew it was the year that your love and passion for aesthetics and perfecting your techniques grew tremendously." I have to give credit to Dr. de Maio for sharing his knowledge and working to divide the face into scientific code sections. I find that using codes to set "the foundation of filler," as he coins it in his training, is a MUST!

If you're looking to up your game in full-face assessment and vertical restoration, I would recommend one of his books or to splurge on an in-person class. This will help you learn all the techniques and nuances that make a noticeable difference in outcomes.

Another trainer to watch is Katie Bader, PA-C. She possesses great insight into how to inject, especially in the midface. I have personally learned a lot from her and highly recommend her trainings.

Jawline

It didn't seem like people were talking about jawlines and chins years ago. Yet looking back at movie stars in old black-and-white films, they all had a beautiful jawline. It's just that no one was talking about it—probably because it was an area of the body that we couldn't easily change. These days, there's so much we can do to reshape the jaw, which makes a major difference in the face's appearance overall—especially the profile.

For both men and women, having a strong jawline that comes forward and aligns vertically is the current aesthetic zeitgeist. Many young people today are acutely aware of this, and they stick their lower jaw out whenever they pose for a photo or selfie. Some have even taken to mewing, a scientifically unproven technique that involves pressing the tongue against the roof of the mouth in an attempt to better define the jawline. These days, even orthodontists have ventured into reshaping retrognathic jawlines in order to bring the bottom jaw forward. Young people who get braces could end up having a real advantage with their jawline in this regard!

I recently attended an aesthetics conference in Beverly Hills where we talked at length about how much jaw shape matters. For men, a wide, square, masculine jawline is associated with power and influence. (Think Brad Pitt and Elon Musk!) The ideal angle looks like a hockey stick when measured from the ear. Male college students who have this type of strong jawline are proven to have more girlfriends and more sex than male students who have a weaker jawline.[70] For women, a clearly defined jawline is also the ideal, albeit with a narrower chin, the perfect bottom point to a feminine, heart-shaped face.

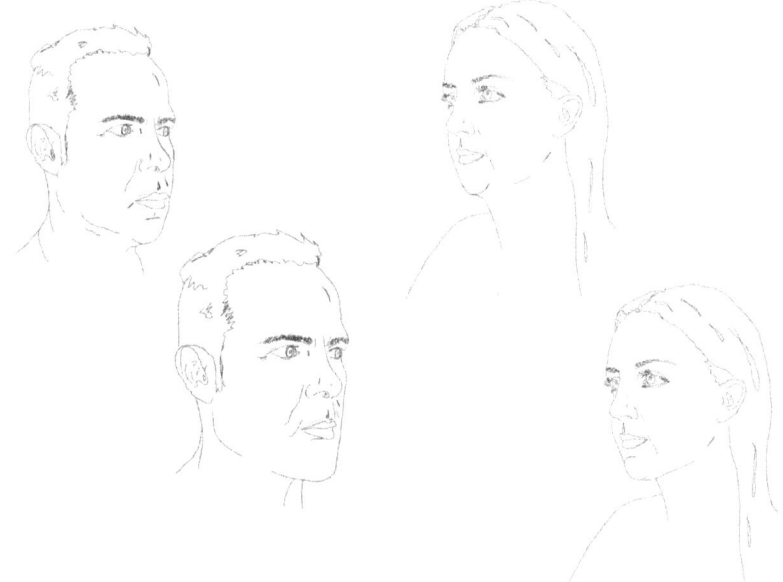

For those of us who weren't lucky enough to have been born with the genetics for a perfect chin or jawline, injecting filler into the chin can work wonders for men or women alike to add more volume where they need it.

Whenever I speak with patients about their jawline, they usually tell me what they don't like rather than specifics on what they would like to achieve. They often complain about having a double chin. When we all started spending more time on Zoom, that was a key observation that many of my middle-aged patients had about their appearance on video. They wanted to know how the bottom of their chin got to be so fat. As we age, we lose bone mass in the jawline, which can create the effect of fullness underneath the chin. We are not gaining fat there but rather changing the ratio of bone to fat. Instead of trying to get rid of some of this volume, it's amazing what a little bit of Juvéderm Volux can do! Adding volume to the jawline can help recreate a sharp edge that decreases the appearance of a double chin.

This can also help women achieve a sharper-looking jawline. As we age, our mentalis muscle builds up from underlying bone loss. The result can be a wider, more square-shaped jaw. This happens to the best of us—even Jennifer Aniston! Filler can help define the jawline and make the face look more youthful.

Lips

I have been doing lip filler for two decades, and we have come a long way over the years! I remember when our options weren't great and we were using products that often caused granulomas and an uneven appearance. Goldie Hawn's duck-bill lips in *The First Wives Club* scared many people away from filler, and it's easy to see why. But times have changed, and now there are great options for creating a little "jeuje" in the lips while still looking natural.

In 2006, Juvéderm XC became approved for facial rejuvenation, and it revolutionized the aesthetics space. The consistency is smooth and firm—and it moves easily, which is especially important on a part of the face that has so much movement. The more advanced Juvéderm Ultra XC Lip Filler is a similar product that works wonders for adding volume, hydration, and shape. I love to use it to get a more youthful appearance while remaining natural.

Another great option for lip filler is Volbella, a type of vycross, which came on the market in 2016. I often use this for patients who are in their 40s or older after we have restored volume loss in the temples, midface, and jawline and they want to make their lips look more youthful. As we age, we can get linear lines (smoker's lines) on the upper cutaneous lip. Volbella can act as scaffolding to restore volume and decrease the appearance of these fine lines. The result is subtle and beautiful. I can't remember a time when one of these patients wasn't happy with the outcome.

Skinvive is another smart option for the lips. Rather than being a filler, it's an injectable skin hydration. It was newly approved in the United States but has been popular in Europe for quite a while. It's almost like injecting lip gloss. It does an excellent job of maintaining hydration in the lips, and the price point is appealing. It's a good option for patients who want to make a change but are scared of filler. (Note that Skinvive can be injected all over the face for hydration, but I don't typically recommend it because the results don't seem noticeable enough to go through the pain of so many tiny needle pricks. I tend to use this product on the mid cheeks, the accordion lines of the lower face, and the lips.)

Although we've come a long way when it comes to enhancing the lips, patients often get pushback from their partners about going down this road. A friend of mine was recently in this situation. She told me that she was interested in lip filler but her husband was scared she would end up looking like a duck. I consulted with her and she decided that she wanted to start small and take a stairstep approach. This would enable us to drive small, incremental changes that would be undetectable to those in her social circle. I started out using Skinvive in the lips to improve hydration, and she was impressed by the subtle results. Next, we moved on to Volbella. She absolutely loved the way that turned out! After thinking about getting lip treatments for so many years, she couldn't believe that she'd waited that long! She is elated, and her husband says she looks totally natural—only 10 years younger!

Earlobes

My friend and her husband own a chain of jewelry stores, and we've talked many times about how women want to wear beautiful jewelry but many get to a point where they don't like the appearance of their earlobes. Even with precious gems catching the light, all they can see is crinkly, atrophied skin. My friend gives her customers the option to add the clear discs that go between the back of the ear and the earing back, which help earrings to not droop forward. This can be a good solution, but filler can provide even better results. My favorite one for this area is Vollure because the density is a good match. I have tried Volbella as well, but it doesn't seem to be dense enough for the earlobes of mature patients.

After injecting in this area, I tell patients not to wear earrings for about two weeks. This has not only been a fun area to augment but also a great way to help my older patients feel a little younger.

Under-eyes

As we age, the under-eye area can appear to hollow or look puffy. We call these under-eye bags. But as we age, the ligaments under the eyes become weaker, and it can become a lower-drooping puffiness under the eyes. These are known as "festoons." Volbella is FDA approved to treat this area, and it works well for many patients. Before you treat the under-eyes, it's important to start with Voluma in the midface as it is the scaffolding for the under-eye hollows. Less is more here. I usually use needle on bone for the area lateral and inferior to the eye. For the medial portion, I prefer a cannula.

After this is complete, using Volbella under the eyes can enhance the overall appearance by reducing some of that under-eye shadowing. That said, the results are subtle, and patients need to have realistic expectations.

Not everyone is a candidate for under-eye filler. If the skin is too loose, it won't hold the filler. If patients have that kind of under-eye appearance, do not inject there. Another thing to watch for is when patients have a lot of pigment under their eyes. They aren't great candidates for under-eye filler because with the additional volume, the light will hit that area differently and make it look even darker. It's kind of like how water looks darker when it's deeper. If patients are already starting with darker pigment in that part of the face, it's not recommended to inject there.

Post-care

After providing filler, it is essential to give patients detailed post-care instructions and make sure they understand the importance of following them in order to reduce risks of filler migration and other adverse outcomes. Make sure your patients do the following:

- Icepack: After treatment, to keep the swelling down, ice the area. Also know that the first injections are usually the most painful and additional rounds tend to be easier.
- Exercise: Do not work out for 24 to 48 hours, especially any workouts that involve valsava movements, which are forceful attempts of exhalation against a closed airway.
- Eating: Try to avoid chewing dense foods for the first two days.
- Contact: Do not touch the area with your fingers, phone, or any other object for several hours after the procedure.
- Products: Do not apply makeup or any other skincare product for 12 to 24 hours due to the topical sodium hypochlorite gel that will be applied to the injection sites.
- Heat/sun: Avoid heat and sun exposure for 24 hours.
- Teeth: Make sure you do not have dental work performed on you 2 to 4 weeks before or after filler. (This is something we recently added due to new research.[71])
- Sleep: If filler has been applied to the midface or jawline, sleep only on your back for the next 24 hours.
- Watching for adverse reactions: Watch for signs of vascular occlusion such as a tender, rapidly expanding bruise, white pustules, or any signs of a stroke. Contact your practitioner's emergency line or go to the emergency room if there are any concerns.

How to make filler last longer

Filler is designed to last for a certain length of time, depending on the product and where it's injected. For example, Voluma has been proven to last in the midface for 24 months with optimal treatment. I've found that you can extend this period if you inject a smaller amount again at, say, a year and a half. This is a good trick for patients who want to make the most out of their injections. If you wait until filler is totally gone, it's like you're working from scratch. Katie Bader advised going until about three-quarters of the way through the expected life and then injecting more. This has worked well for me personally, as well as for my patients.

Plan for adverse outcomes

Safety is always the top priority in aesthetic medicine. There are inherently going to be risks in any treatment, but the risks for filler are greater than for other types of treatments. Filler is an implantable device. It's a serious medical procedure.

As a practitioner, you must be trained on how to handle adverse outcomes, and you must have a plan. As mentioned in chapter 2 with Dr. Downie, the biggest concern when injecting filler is having a vascular occlusion.

Julie Bass Kaplan, NP, understands this risk very well. Her journey into aesthetics took a dramatic turn in February 2010 when, while receiving filler from a trainer, she noticed something alarming: a blanching effect that caused her skin to turn white and then blue. This was the beginning of a vascular occlusion. Back then, however, few people in the aesthetics world recognized the signs, let alone had a protocol for dealing with it.

Julie's reaction worsened quickly, with her face becoming necrotic, developing sores, and ultimately causing significant damage to her skin.[72] With no standard procedures or established guidelines at that time, Julie and her husband, a facial plastic surgeon, scrambled to try everything they could to save her skin. From massaging the area with heat to adding oxygen and taking aspirin, they were forced to improvise. It was a harrowing experience—but one that ignited Julie's passion for creating safety protocols to prevent others from going through the same ordeal.

At a time when hyaluronidase (the enzyme used to dissolve hyaluronic-acid-based fillers) wasn't readily available, Julie had to be resourceful. She was determined to pioneer change, and she did. Over the years, she developed protocols that became industry standards, sharing her knowledge freely with others. Her experience spurred her to help other practitioners and patients avoid the potentially devastating effects of filler complications. She is now a passionate advocate for safety in aesthetic treatments, regularly conducting mock drills with her team and training others on the best practices for treating occlusions.

Develop a vascular occlusion protocol

The question is not *if* you're going to have a vascular occlusion but *when*. That's because there are vessels and arteries under the skin that you can't see with the naked eye. Consider them little invisible land mines. If you inject into or too close to them, you can restrict or block blood flow, which can lead to tissue damage or, in severe cases, necrosis or blindness. Facial veins and arteries vary when it comes to individual anatomy. I only learned last year how much variability there is when it comes to the location of foramens (small openings) people have on their face, each one a center for vessels and nerves. People can have six on one side and one on the other. It can vary by continent and race as well. Oftentimes you can feel them and know where to avoid, but not always.

It's important to understand how tricky this is so that you're well aware of the risks and prepared to handle any adverse outcomes. Even if you've been injecting for years, you can still hit a vessel.

That's why the number-one thing to do is to develop a protocol for handling vascular occlusions. The literature is constantly evolving, so stay current on new research and best practices. I have been using the 2021 American Society of Dermatologic Surgery task-force paper at my practice, along with other research. I encourage you to look this up and use it as a basis for your own protocol, adding other steps as needed.[73] Here are a couple highlights from our protocol:

- Always monitor for blanching or skin whitening when injecting. If this lasts a few seconds or more, stop injecting and massage the area until it returns to a normal color. If normal skin coloring does not return, do not continue with the injection.
- In case of a true occlusion, hyaluronidase injection should be done immediately along with skin massage. Intralesional or systemic corticosteroids can also be used. Use warm compresses and oral aspirin.
- Track the expiration date of your hyaluronidase and make sure you order more before you need it so that your emergency kit is always up to date. This is a small price to pay for keeping your patients safe.
- Do drills with your team so everyone knows what to do in case of an emergency.

In my practice, we have our protocol typed up and in an emergency kit. We have two versions—our traditional protocol and the blindness protocol—from which we use the ophthalmic literature.

Develop a blindness protocol

Blindness can occur from the ophthalmic artery being occluded. It is a rare side effect that must be addressed immediately. You will only have about eight minutes before a patient will permanently lose their vision, so you must have a solid plan in place for handling this—and you need to practice this plan. Otherwise, there's no way you'll be able to deal with such an emergency in time to save a patient's vision.

If a patient mentions any change in vision, immediately do a quick visual acuity assessment. This includes 1) the ability to read letters, count fingers, and perceive hand motions; 2) light perception; 3) extraocular muscle function; and 4) papillary response to light.

If the patient confirms any change in vision, you need to switch into the fastest gear you possibly have and transfer them to a hospital or ophthalmologist equipped to help with this situation.

In my practice, we have an ophthalmology department we collaborate with for this. I had a session during which a doctor walked us through retrobulbar (behind the eyeball) injections just so I'd know what to do if we were unable to get to them in time. I strongly hope that I never need to put this knowledge into practice, since that department is just up the street from us, but I am prepared to do so if necessary.

If you haven't contacted an ophthalmologist to partner with in case of emergency, this is your sign that it's time to do so. Once you have a plan in place, do a drill. See how long it takes you to provide the right treatment and adjust as needed to improve safety precautions.

Know how and when to dissolve filler

Good filler is both tasteful and undetectable. After the initial swelling goes down, patients should look a bit younger and fresher than when they came in. But sometimes outcomes do not align with expectations. Instead of looking younger, patients can look puffy or swollen, which can become apparent in the weeks following the treatment. Maybe too much filler was injected or it wasn't placed as well as it could have been. This happens all the time, even to celebrities such as Kylie Jenner and Madonna.

Another tricky factor here is migration. Although fillers are designed to stay in the location where they are injected, this doesn't happen perfectly. Instead, fillers move and spread over time. Many factors affect the way this happens, including the type of filler and viscosity, the way it's injected, how much is injected, a patient's unique anatomy, and the natural movement of their facial muscles. With proper technique, practitioners can plan for migration and control it well, but sometimes filler behaves in unexpected ways. This can create an uneven, unnatural, or unflattering appearance—either in the weeks following treatment or months later.

If this happens to one of your patients, the most important thing is for everyone to stay calm and work toward a solution together. Remember that filler isn't permanent. Aside from it dissolving naturally over time, it can be manually dissolved with hyaluronidase.

Not all practitioners who inject filler know how to dissolve it. I am acutely aware of this because I get a lot of patients at my office who want help dissolving filler that other practitioners injected. If you aren't comfortable dissolving filler, it's time to learn. Ask the rep who sells you your filler if they know of any good training courses, or check with your academy. Julie Bass Kaplan's training is a great option as well. In the meantime, make sure you help your patients find someone who can treat them.

Find your village

When one of your patients is having an issue, it helps to have other experts to consult with. One time, a patient contacted our emergency line the day after she'd gotten filler because she was experiencing symptoms that were potentially filler related, including a racing heart and headache. I looped in my trainer, Katie Bader, and she looped in her colleague, Nicola Lowrey. After telling them the symptoms, they thought the patient might just be experiencing an anxiety attack. Katie told me to ask the patient if she was feeling nervous. The patient said she was feeling very anxious and was unable to think of anything but the risk of a vascular occlusion. After we talked for about five minutes, the patient was able to calm down, and we all realized that everything was OK. Sometimes it takes a village! Get a Katie or a Nicola in your network to help when you need it, and make sure you pay it forward to other practitioners as well. There are times when we all need a little support.

Out of all the aesthetic treatments available today, I'd say that fillers have revolutionized aesthetic medicine the most by offering a minimally invasive way to restore volume, enhance contours, and rejuvenate the face. However, achieving optimal results requires not just a deep understanding of facial anatomy but also a commitment to precision and safety. As with any aesthetic treatment, fillers are an art form. Your skill and knowledge are key to crafting natural, balanced results.

Personally, fillers have kept me excited about the aesthetics field over the years. There is always something to learn because the science evolves so quickly—and there's so much nuance to ensuring that each patient's unique features are respected and enhanced with care. I encourage you to lean into this and continue deepening your expertise so that you can provide the best possible experience for your patients.

CHAPTER 10

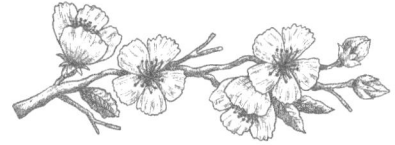

The Skinny on Weight-Loss Treatments

For many of us, being able to target specific areas for fat loss sounds like a dream! Losing weight isn't easy, especially as we age. Diet and exercise can be a grueling journey that doesn't always lead to ideal results. In a society that values thinness, carrying extra fat can be one of the key drivers of low self-esteem. In aesthetics, we have a variety of treatments that can help slim and smooth.

However, it hasn't always been this way. It was not that long ago when, relatively speaking, large, curvy bodies were the goal. I remember being in a second-floor classroom in Avignon, France, during one of our first days of art history listening to my professor, Monsieur Hervé, cite how beautiful the large, curvy women were in the Renaissance paintings. I thought that my French was inadequate and that I wasn't translating very well. Turns out I was hearing him correctly. I just didn't realize that it used to be en vogue to have a thicker body. This was the 1990s and the fad was very-skinny supermodels.

During this time, a controversial song by Sir Mix-a-Lot challenged this notion when he proclaimed, "I like big butts, and I cannot lie." This song started shock waves of culture change. Part of the controversy was the mention of buttocks in a sexual manner in general (it was briefly banned on MTV), but another part of the controversy was that it went against the aesthetic zeitgeist of the time.[74] Women were getting mixed messaging. Should they aim to be "heroin chic" or should they embrace a curvaceous figure?

During the Renaissance, having a curvaceous body was idealized because it meant you had the ability to feed yourself due to your financial status. It wasn't until the turn of the century and 1920s flapper era that the aesthetic preferences changed to a thinner silhouette, with women wearing much smaller outfits and taping down their breasts. The new aesthetic was to be thin, indicating that you were wealthy enough to not only afford food but choose not to eat. This marked the beginning of dieting culture. Interestingly, this was also right around the time that the bathroom scale (patented in 1916) became popular.[75] Since then, society has always had some level of interest in staying slim.

I spoke with Dr. Spencer Berry, who is board certified in obesity medicine and has been on the national board of directors for the National Obesity Medical Association. He's been caring for overweight patients for decades. He became interested in this area of medicine when he found that if most of his patients could lose 10 percent of their body weight, a lot of their diseases (e.g., hypertension, heart disease, and diabetes) would go away. He felt called to help patients make that progress.

Dr. Berry believes that health is a combination of physical, mental, emotional, and psychological factors. To help overweight or obese patients reach a healthier weight—and maintain it—he encourages looking at how each of these factors plays a role. He says that when patients feel better physically, they often feel better mentally, and vice versa. It's all tied together, and improvement creates a virtuous cycle.

This is such an important insight for all of us in aesthetics. Even though we have the power to make some enhancements to a person's weight or shape with today's treatments, it isn't magic. If there are underlying issues that are leading to continued weight gain, such as depression or unhealthy habits, the way to make real progress is by addressing those head-on, just as Dr. Berry did.

Not only is Dr. Berry an expert in obesity medicine, but he also helps patients across the continuum of their weight-loss journey by also addressing how fat loss affects the face. A downside to slimming down that a lot of people don't consider is that when you lose fat, you lose it all over your body—including your face. When you're younger, the collagen and elastin can snap back. But when you're older, it doesn't work that way. You can lose weight and feel great about your body, but your face can appear to be saggy and hollow. The older you are and more weight you lose, the bigger the problem.

Dr. Berry got involved in aesthetics and volume replacement (filler) of the face because so many patients were experiencing this issue and bringing it to his attention. Knowing how important it is for patients to feel good about themselves, he began working with patients to proactively help them address skin quality as they lose weight.

This sounds so simple and logical, but only a small percentage of weight-loss patients are getting this kind of holistic support. Unfortunately, most patients don't realize that they should be thinking about aesthetics until after it's too late. They are so excited about shedding pounds that they don't notice the minor changes in their face that make them look older. The rise of the weight-loss drug Ozempic is exponentially increasing the number of people who are dealing with this issue, now coined "Ozempic face." After losing a massive amount of weight quickly, patients are unhappy with their hollow cheeks, sunken eyes, more prominent jowls, increased wrinkles, and sagging skin. Although aesthetic treatments can address these issues, it's not easy. A better approach is to focus on prevention through treatments while the body is transforming.

I recommend serial laser treatments during a patient's weight-loss journey so they can rejuvenate and thicken the collagen and keep it tighter. If skin quality is better while they are shedding pounds, it will snap back better when they reach their ideal weight. Fillers can also be used to help add volume where needed and prevent excess sagging. For patients who are highly concerned about their skin quality, there could also be a strong argument for losing weight at a more gradual pace to give skin more time to respond to aesthetic treatments.

Liposuction

For patients who have struggled for many years with weight loss, liposuction could be an option, but like any surgery, it comes with risks. About one in 5,000 people die on the table or from complications.[76] A high-profile example of this is Donda West, Kanye West's mother, who died the day after getting liposuction, a tummy tuck, and a breast reduction in 2007.[77] Even with successful lipo procedures, the results oftentimes aren't perfect. Skin dimpling is a common result, especially on the legs. However, some plastic surgeons have found that radio-frequency treatments can tighten the skin directly after liposuction and therefore have improved outcomes. Lipo is also prohibitively expensive for many people. If people can lose weight without going under the knife, that's typically a much better option.

Fat freezing

The discovery of fat freezing has an interesting origin story rooted in observations made by doctors about the effects of cold on fat cells. One of the key anecdotes involves women who rode horses in cold weather. The first published study was in the 1980s.[78] They noticed that their thighs became slimmer over time, even though they weren't specifically trying to lose fat. How could this happen? Were their muscles somehow working extra hard to burn the fat? Doctors finally realized that it was due to the friction and pressure from riding, combined with the cold temperatures. This suggested that prolonged exposure to cold could target and reduce fat deposits.

This observation was linked to another interesting discovery. In the 1970s, doctors began to notice a phenomenon called "popsicle panniculitis," wherein children who ate popsicles developed dimples in their cheeks. This was due to the cold from the popsicles causing fat loss in the area.

These observations led researchers to think that cold might selectively reduce fat without damaging the surrounding skin and tissues. This eventually inspired the development of cryolipolysis, a non-invasive procedure that uses controlled cooling to target and eliminate fat cells without harming the surrounding tissue. The procedure, now commonly known as CoolSculpting, was developed in the early 2000s by scientists at Harvard University, building on these early insights.

Taking a look at this a little differently, another modality that has the same outcome is Kybella (the brand name for deoxycholic acid), a naturally occurring molecule in the body that aids in the breakdown and absorption of dietary fat. Kybella is injected directly into the submental fat (the fat under the chin). Once injected, it works by breaking down the cell membrane of fat cells, effectively destroying them. This process is called lipolysis. The destroyed fat cells are no longer able to store or accumulate fat and, over time, the body naturally metabolizes and eliminates these dead cells through its normal waste-removal processes. As this happens, the treated area gradually becomes slimmer and more contoured.

Fat freezing can help patients achieve noticeable results, but they need to know what to expect with the results. The best candidates for fat freezing are patients who are close to or at their ideal weight and desire a small amount of fat reduction or smoothing of the skin in specific areas.

Rather than looking at fat freezing as a real weight-loss option, it makes more sense to view it as a way to subtly change the shape of the body. If a person doesn't like how their stomach pooches out under their belly button after having had a couple kids, the way their outer thighs give their body more of a pear shape than an hourglass shape, addressing these concerns could be realistic goals for CoolSculpting. If a person wants to change how their chin slopes downward into their neck, Kybella could make a noticeable difference.

Personally, I've tried both and enjoyed the results. When we first got a CoolSculpting machine at my clinic, my colleagues and I were so excited! After doing the proper training for using the machine, we couldn't wait to try it out!

We practiced on each other, using it on the inner thighs, flanks, and abdomen. We have definitely gotten better at this modality over the years, and I find it especially helpful in two areas: the submental fat and the upper arms. Show me a woman past menopause who doesn't have excess adipose tissue in these areas.[79] (My mother used to teasingly call her drooping upper arms "angel wings" when she hugged her grandchildren, but she would have definitely wanted CoolSculpting to treat this area if it had been an option while she was alive and healthy.)

I think fat freezing can be a game changer for those areas where it's particularly difficult to lose weight. I was just scrolling through Facebook and saw a comment come up in my Physician Mom Group posted by a doctor who was asking her plastics and dermatology colleagues how to reduce her uneven buttocks. Nuances in shape bother a lot of people despite their body weight.

It typically takes a few sessions before CoolSculpting will yield any noticeable results, but we have been pleased to notice that it makes a lasting difference. And when it comes to Kybella, I've personally had injections under my chin on a few different occasions, and I've always been pleased with the results. That's one area of the body where you can't do targeted exercises, so it's nice to have a treatment option that makes a real difference.

Fat freezing has grown in popularity over the past several years, but it's also seen a few hiccups along the way. A very high-profile example of this is when former supermodel Linda Evangelista got CoolSculpting all over her body from 2015 to 2016 and ended up being in the less than 1 percent of patients who experience adverse outcomes. Although, the vast majority of the time, fat-freezing treatments are effective in reducing fat, sometimes patients experience the opposite—paradoxical adipose hyperplasia (PH)—wherein fatty tissue thickens and expands. Imagine the horror of gaining additional fat in the exact areas where you wanted to lose it! This is what happened to Evangelista. She withdrew from the public eye and sued the maker of CoolSculpting (which at the time was Zeltiq Aesthetics) for $50 million. They settled out of court for an undisclosed amount.[80] The ordeal was quite public, and it was terrible press for CoolSculpting.

This is unfortunate, especially since the issue could likely have been avoided if Evangelista had only done a small amount of the treatment in one area of her body to test it and then waited to see if she experienced any negative symptoms. This is always a best practice for any type of treatment or product as bad reactions do happen. With this in mind, it's essential to know how long you need to wait before assessing the success of the procedure. Evangelista's lawsuit cited seven sessions of CoolSculpting at her dermatologist's office over the course of about seven months. This shows that it could take up to seven months to identify symptoms of PH. That's a long time! Practitioners must be aware of this when they advise patients of the risks. It's also helpful to know that, today, CoolSculpting (now owned by Allergan) offers up to $7,500 in compensation for patients who get PH so that they can get their treatment covered.

All this information is enough to scare a lot of patients away from CoolSculpting, even though the risk is less than 1 percent. I still feel confident that it is a solid treatment choice when administered responsibly and cautiously. Luckily, for those who feel differently, there are other options.

Why can't we take an ice pack and melt off our fat at home?

Wouldn't it be easy to just sit in front of the TV, rub some ice packs on our thighs, and wait for the magic to happen? Unfortunately, there are several reasons why that won't work. Cryolipolysis, the process used in professional fat-freezing treatments such as CoolSculpting, requires precise and controlled cooling to target fat cells. The devices themselves are calibrated to cool the fat to a specific temperature that triggers fat-cell death (apoptosis) without harming the surrounding tissues such as skin, nerves, and muscles. Cold packs from your freezer aren't capable of maintaining the precise temperature and consistency needed for this process. Additionally, professional cryolipolysis devices are designed to reach and affect the subcutaneous fat layer, specifically. Cold packs, on the other hand, primarily affect the skin and superficial layers of tissue. They do not penetrate deeply enough to effectively reach and target fat cells. Lastly, applying ice or cold packs directly to the skin for extended periods can cause frostbite or cold burns. Without the protective measures and controlled environment of a professional treatment, you risk damaging your skin and underlying tissues.

This is the issue with cryogenic tanks and ice baths where you submerge the whole body to stimulate fat loss. These are unproven from a scientific perspective. Although many people swear by them, it's important to be aware of the risks.

CoolSculpting vs. Kybella

Many people wonder which one they should use and why. This is an excellent question! If you approach this wrong, it can be a missed opportunity for driving the best outcomes.

At the time of this writing, Kybella is only approved for use under the chin. That said, I have used it off-label on other areas as well, including saddlebags that are too small for CoolSculpting and irregularities of the abdomen.

CoolSculpting and Kybella used to be different companies. Now they are the same: Allergan. Today, Allergan has good training protocols and is getting the message out there that the right order should be CoolSculpting and then Kybella. Of course, figuring this out took trial and error!

When Kybella first came out, a friend of mine who works in the aesthetics space jumped in and had it done right away under her chin. As many practitioners in the industry do, we have relatively fast and easy access to these tools, and we often use them on ourselves and our colleagues! It's a fun perk to have access to new technology, but it also means we treat ourselves as guinea pigs to some degree through experimentation.

My friend had several sessions of Kybella but could not seem to get rid of the submental fat under her chin. She finally realized the issue: she needed to debulk *first*. She therefore tried CoolSculpting. To her surprise, it didn't work. She realized then that the Kybella could have caused some fibrosis (scarring in the skin) from the acid, which made the area not responsive to CoolSculpting.

The lesson? If a patient has enough fat for CoolSculpting, it's important to do that treatment first and then fine-tune with Kybella.

The CoolSculpting machine comes with a piece that fits on a patient's neck. You should always use this to determine how to move forward. Eyeballing the volume in a patient's chin can be deceiving because even people who are thin can have excess fat under the chin. Sometimes it's just genetics! If there's enough fat to fill the CoolSculpting piece, the patient is a good candidate for CoolSculpting and they should start with that area. After they lose volume there, which could take multiple sessions, they would then move on to Kybella for fine-tuning, if desired. If they don't have enough fat to fill the CoolSculpting piece, they should skip that step and be a candidate for Kybella if they have unwanted fat under their chin.

How to use fat freezing

Here are some of my best tips and tricks for fat freezing.

Document: I recommend taking detailed before-and-after photos. We use a rotating platform in our office, provided by CoolSculpting, with a solid background behind the patient. It is very important that consistent photos be taken so we can do proper analysis for our patients. You can also use 3-D imaging to see exactly how a person's shape changes over time with the treatments.

Neck/jawline: Results typically become noticeable after a few weeks, with full effects visible after a few months. Since the fat cells are destroyed and eliminated, the results of Kybella and CoolSculpting are considered permanent. However, maintaining a stable weight is important as remaining fat cells can still expand with weight gain.

Note that we never target the face for fat loss. To maintain a youthful appearance, we want to add volume in the face, not take it away. That is why rapid weight loss with GLP-1 medications has led to such a characteristic face: Ozempic face.

Butt: Some patients have uneven buttocks inferiorly or laterally and often need sculpting of these areas with precision fat freezing. But be careful to make sure you are on the same page as your patient. Note that the mini applicator might need to be used in this area.

Thighs: How many women do you know who have lateral thighs that fit the characteristic "saddlebags"? I think it's fair to say that most women don't love having this look. The applicators for this area are specially designed for the curvature here and help to better define the transition area between the buttocks and thighs.

As for the inner thighs, Allergan had to switch up the CoolSculpting applicator and use a straight panel to avoid scalloping of the fat that was produced early on with the curved applicator. The applicator now avoids this feature.

Abdomen: The muffin top in this area is a frustrating protuberance that often remains despite weight loss and diet changes. Most practitioners usually use the curved applicator; however, in patients who have a hernia or are sensitive, a flat panel may be a better option. In my family, several of us on one side have a genetic predisposition to umbilical hernias, especially after childbirth. I didn't want to miss out on CoolSculpting in this area, so we researched this and found that if a flat panel, such as for the inner thighs, was used, it was safe.

Above the knee: It's also possible to reduce fat in the area above the knee, although this is currently off-label. For this area, if we were to treat it, we would use the mini applicator that is used for the submental fat.

Focus on symmetry: Achieving symmetry can be difficult and time-consuming for practitioners. It's essential to pay very close attention to what you're doing on one side of the body so that you can do the same on the other side. It's also possible that a patient's body isn't symmetrical, in which case you'll need to adjust by doing something slightly different on one side so that you achieve symmetry in the results. We have found that if we have the patient look at our drawings of where the applicators will be applied and they agree about the plan ahead of time, positive realistic outcomes are higher.

After-care: If patients are noticing pain after their CoolSculpting, an ice pack can be helpful. The first 1 to 2 days are often the most sensitive. Patients should be instructed to take good care of themselves after treatment.

Electromagnetic muscle stimulation

Losing fat is great, but to look good in a swimsuit, being toned helps a lot too! There are a couple of popular muscle-building devices on the market. Let's focus on Emsculpt and CoolTone. They both use magnetic fields to achieve their outcomes. Emsculpt was introduced to the market in 2018 as a way to develop muscles without exercising, using a technology called high-intensity focused electromagnetic (HIFEM) energy. This energy induces powerful muscle contractions that are much more intense than what can be achieved through voluntary exercise. During an Emsculpt session, the targeted muscles undergo thousands of supramaximal contractions in a short period. These are involuntary contractions that are significantly stronger and more rapid than typical muscle contractions during exercise. The intense contractions cause the muscle fibers to remodel themselves. This involves an increase in the number of muscle fibers (muscle hyperplasia) and the size of existing muscle fibers (muscle hypertrophy). Essentially, the muscles adapt by growing stronger and larger, similar to what happens after strength-training exercises. The result is increased muscle mass and improved muscle tone in the treated area. Common areas treated with Emsculpt include the abdomen, buttocks, thighs, arms, and calves.

A typical Emsculpt session lasts about 30 minutes, and multiple sessions are usually recommended for optimal results. Most treatment plans involve four sessions spaced over a two-week period. Patients typically start seeing visible results after a few weeks, with continued improvement over the following months. The full effects are usually seen around two to four weeks after the final session. To maintain results, some patients may choose to have periodic maintenance treatments, especially if they are not regularly engaging in muscle-strengthening exercises.

Emsculpt is ideal for individuals who are already relatively fit and are looking to enhance muscle tone and reduce stubborn fat pockets. It's not a weight-loss solution but rather a body-contouring treatment. Emsculpt is popular among those seeking a non-surgical way to sculpt their body, particularly in areas where building muscle and reducing fat through traditional exercise and diet may be challenging. It's a great option for achieving a more toned and defined physique without surgery or downtime. It also claims some fat reduction with the muscle building.

CoolTone is very similar and uses magnetic muscle stimulation (MMS) technology, which also stimulates muscle contractions but with a slightly different frequency and depth. The sessions are similar in length and protocol. The main difference is that MMS focuses solely on strengthening and toning muscles through muscle stimulation and is potentially more intense with the technology focused only on muscle toning without fat reduction.

Looking toward the future

Weight loss is a highly personal and emotional journey. I struggled with it for many years. I was doing intermittent fasting, but it wasn't really making an impact. At one point, I tried supplements and herbs—and I actually gained more weight! On top of that, I felt a little off. I started getting lightheaded, had trouble sleeping. I felt fatigued, and it seemed like my pulse would spike higher than it should out of nowhere.

Even though I'm a doctor, I realized that I needed help from another doctor that specializes in weight loss. I ended up going to the Mayo Clinic. They told me that many supplements are contaminated with other ingredients and that this was likely the cause of me feeling a little off. My doctor recommended that I stop taking the supplements and try diet and exercise. My local primary-care doctor then recommended intermittent fasting. I told her that I was already fasting, but when she pointed out the details about how to do it properly, I realized that I'd been doing it wrong. It turns out that if you eat anything during your fasting window, even a zero-calorie sweetener, your brain thinks food is coming and signals your body to start making insulin. This can cause you to feel shaky (hypoglycemic) and make it harder to finish the fasting. The cream in my coffee was breaking my fast, and worse, the gum I constantly chewed was "turning on" my pancreas and making my body think I was eating. So even though I had abstained from food for many hours a day for years, it was futile because I wasn't fully fasting. I stopped having cream in my coffee and I switched from gum to mints. I lost 18 pounds in about a year and a half without making any other changes. That was a big win for me.

There are so many nuances to weight loss! Little strategies can add up and make a big difference. That's why it's so important to get personalized care from a primary-care doctor—and even better, a specialist. This is what I tell all my patients who are interested in losing weight.

As aesthetic practitioners, we play an important role in holistic care, but we're only one spoke in the wheel.

We are at an interesting point in time when it comes to weight loss. Science and technology are advancing exponentially, and the options for shedding pounds are becoming better than ever before. Though the jury is still out on the long-term side effects of Ozempic, as aesthetic practitioners, we can't ignore how it's entered the market. One in eight adults in the United States has tried a GLP-1 drug.[81] As more people look to Ozempic or similar GLP-1 medications for support losing a significant amount of fat, the demand for both liposuction and fat freezing is decreasing. It's safe to say that people will always want help enhancing the nuances of their shape, so I don't expect Ozempic to kill these parts of the market. But it's definitely a trend to keep an eye on. At the same time, as we see an increase in the number of people losing a significant amount of weight, we can expect more and more patients who seek support for skin-tightening treatments—especially on the face. This is certainly an opportunity for practitioners to position their services and expertise to meet future demands in the market.

CHAPTER 11

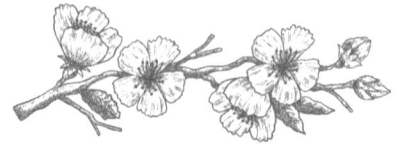

Radiofrequency

Radiofrequency (RF) is a non-invasive option for reducing the appearance of fine lines, wrinkles, and sagging skin. It is often referred to as the "nonsurgical facelift," but RF isn't just for the face. Treatments can work well all over the body, including the neck, legs, buttocks, abdomen, or wherever patients want to increase firmness or decrease cellulite.

RF works by using electromagnetic waves to heat the deeper layers of the skin, specifically targeting the dermis and subcutaneous tissues. This controlled heat stimulates collagen and elastin production, which are essential proteins for maintaining skin firmness and elasticity. As a result, skin looks tighter and smoother.

It's interesting how this works, since the temperature of the RF machine is only between 106 and 110°F, or 41 and 43°C. That's because RF generates heat as a result of different tissue resistance or impedance to the electromagnetic current. This means heat is produced when the tissues' inherent resistance converts the electrical current to thermal energy, as dictated by Ohm's law:

Energy (J) = Current^2 × Resistance × Time[82]

For example, adipose tissue has a high tissue impedance and will generate more heat than muscle, which has lower impedance.[83] In fact, when RF energy is directed to subdermal adipose tissue, it has been shown to generate temperatures seven times higher than those generated by the dermis, which allows RF to kill fat cells without damaging the skin.[84,85] It also tightens the collagen by cleaving the hydrogen bonds in the collagen triple helix, which causes shortening and thickening of the collagen fibrils. However, to ensure this happens, it is important to heat the tissue adequately and test often with the RF machine's thermometer probe.

To clarify, when people talk about RF today, they are often referring to combining radiofrequency with microneedling, which is an invasive cosmetic procedure. It uses small needles plus the radiofrequency to have a more dramatic decrease in wrinkles and fine lines while tightening the skin. However, the RF stand-alone still has benefits when used as the protocol recommends.

One of the major benefits of RF treatments is that they require little to no downtime, allowing people to resume their daily activities immediately after each procedure. That said, when a treatment is less invasive and has less downtime, the results are often less impressive. I've found this to be the case with radiofrequency. Patients need to come in for multiple sessions, and they must understand that results aren't permanent. As long as that is made clear to patients up front and they understand what they're signing up for, results can align with expectations.

A friend of mine had an issue with this recently when she got an RF treatment done in Chicago to treat mild cellulite on her thighs and buttocks. She works out regularly and is at her ideal weight, but as we all know, sometimes cellulite just doesn't want to go away on its own. She told me that the treatment took about 30 minutes, and aside from a couple quick zings, it didn't hurt.

My friend wasn't sure what kind of results to expect. A few hours after the treatment, she looked in the mirror and was shocked. The dimples were completely gone! She went to bed ecstatic about the results, picturing herself finally walking down the beach with confidence. When she woke up in the morning and checked out her backside in the mirror, all the cellulite was back. Not even 24 hours later, she looked exactly like she did before the treatment.

This experience is pretty common, and patients need to be prepped for it or they won't be happy. Initial results are typically noticeable the same day as treatment but wear off quickly, and final results can take a few months. Having patients come in for multiple sessions will yield better results over time. As a patient, the experience can be kind of a roller coaster, with immediate gratification followed quickly by disappointment. That said, the overall appearance of the skin should improve over several months of treatment. After that, people often find that results begin to wear off a year or two later, depending on their skin's starting point, the number of treatments, and the location on the body.

RF can yield good outcomes if done properly, but it takes a lot of patience and diligence on behalf of the practitioner as the device must be stroked back and forth across each area of the skin numerous times. In my experience, it typically takes about seven passes. It's not a quick process—or a particularly interesting treatment for practitioners to provide. On top of that, it can be hard to keep track of which areas of the body have already been treated and how many times. You really do need to have a good approach and lots of patience—and pay attention to what you're doing, or else you might breeze through it too quickly.

Aside from proper technique, the RF machine must be heated to the right temperature range. This is key for ensuring the production of collagen in the skin's dermis layer. If the machine isn't heated high enough, the results won't be as noticeable or last as long. If it's too hot, patients can get burned.

In terms of adding RF as a service option on your aesthetics menu, purchasing an RF machine is not a huge up-front investment, especially compared with other aesthetic treatments. And the amount of training needed to become good at providing RF is certainly less than other services, but it still requires attention and patience.

RF can be a good fit for your patients who can't handle pain and/or don't want anything invasive. If they're willing to come in multiple times for treatment, it can be a good option. Compared with fat-freezing methodologies, treatments are typically less risky and less expensive, which can increase the appeal as well.

Another great selling point with RF is the immediate results it yields. If a person has an important event and wants to look their best for a short period of time, getting an RF treatment can be like waving a magic wand. (Think award shows, performances, photo shoots.) But just like Cinderella at the ball, the magic can wear off quickly. This makes RF the perfect fit for only a certain segment of people and circumstances.

CHAPTER 12

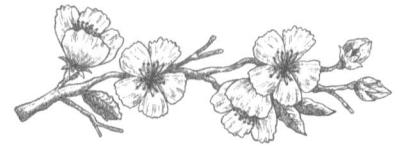

Microneedling, Plasma-Rich Protein, and Exosomes

People have been puncturing their skin for health or cosmetic reasons for thousands of years. Ancient Indian Ayurvedic practices included the use of sharp instruments or fine needles to prick the skin for therapeutic and cosmetic purposes.[86] These methods were believed to help release toxins, improve blood circulation, and promote healthier, more radiant skin. And of course, acupuncture, which dates back over 2,000 years in traditional Chinese medicine and is still popular today, involves inserting fine needles into the skin at specific points in order to balance the body's energy (qi) and promote healing.[87]

Though modern microneedling is a relatively recent development, the underlying concept of using needles or abrasive tools to stimulate skin renewal has been practiced in various forms throughout history. The various methods for creating controlled skin injury to promote healing and enhance beauty can be seen as early precursors to the microneedling techniques used today.

Thanks to modern science, we have a much better understanding of how and why microneedling works for aesthetic purposes: the micro injuries that trigger the body's natural healing processes stimulate collagen and elastin production, which are essential for maintaining firm, youthful skin. This improves skin texture, and tone, while reducing the appearance of fine lines, wrinkles, scars, enlarged pores, and hyperpigmentation (dark patches).

Although most microneedling is done on the face, it can also be used for rejuvenating the skin on the neck and décolletage (the upper chest), areas that often show signs of aging. Microneedling can be used on other parts of the body as well, such as the abdomen or thighs, to treat stretch marks and/or improve skin texture.

Overall, microneedling has become quite popular, and most full-service aesthetic practitioners today offer it. I've found this to be interesting as many of my patients have been underwhelmed by the results. After hearing so many positive things about it, perhaps their expectations are higher than they should be. As a practitioner, this is important to take note of so that I guide patients to the modalities that will yield the results they desire and help manage expectations for their treatments. During a consultation, my team and I explain that microneedling is a good option for those who want a natural, less-invasive skin rejuvenation treatment that comes with relatively low downtime. Most patients feel an improvement to the texture of their skin and only experience mild redness and swelling for a day or two, which makes it comparatively more manageable than other treatments.

A key benefit to microneedling is it enhances the absorption of either platelets or topical skincare products such as serums containing hyaluronic acid, vitamins, or growth factors. This allows for deeper penetration and more effective results from these products. Personally, I wouldn't recommend microneedling unless it's paired with a growth-factor treatment, such as platelet-rich plasma (PRP), platelet-derived growth factor, or exosomes. Applying these products after microneedling greatly enhances outcomes.

Stamps, pens, or rollers?

Broadly speaking, there are three different types of microneedling devices. The needles on these devices typically range in length from 0.5 to 2.5 millimeters, depending on the treatment goals and the area being treated. One type of device works like a stamp that targets a patch of skin, roughly one by two inches, with about 100 to 150 needles at a time. (The stamp-like application is similar to many laser machines.) Another type of device is a pen that targets a tiny area of skin. The tip of the pen has 9 to 12 needles. The third type of device has a rolling wheel covered in hundreds of needles that's attached to a handle and is rolled across and pressed into the skin.

With all these choices on the market, both patients and practitioners are left to wonder what works best.

Let's rule out the rollers first. They don't offer much control or consistency in terms of pressure, which isn't ideal. Most clinics have replaced them with pens or stamps. Rollers are often marketed to consumers to use at home, but at-home microneedling is never recommended (see the following risks section).

After a great deal of experience with stamps and pens, I prefer the stamping devices by a wide margin because they yield better results, which is what matters most. That said, a lot of my PAs prefer using the pen because it's less painful for the patients and ergonomically easier for them. The pen seems less labor intensive because it's smaller and cordless. The pain level is also a bit lower for patients, which means staff don't have to go through the exercise of numbing patients as routinely. But again, it doesn't work as well as the stamp! I find it odd how often I see microneedling pens advertised from med spas and clinics, since most don't do much. But the marketing seems to be working. Many patients are under the impression that the pens are more modern or effective than the stamping devices. It's true that the pens don't have a cord, and the compact design might look like the next generation of the machine, but the truth is the pens are a cheaper and less sophisticated device. The stamping devices are a bigger investment for aesthetic practitioners, but from a business perspective, it's worth it not only due to the results but also because it's so much quicker to use than a pen. When you're able to create 100 to 150 punctures at once instead of 9 to 13, it obviously goes much quicker, and also more uniformly. To be fair, with stamping, sometimes topical numbing—even compounded with higher levels of anesthetic—is not enough for certain patients. In this case, consider adding Pro-Nox to your practice.

Rough costs of microneedling machines

Most companies don't make their pricing public. They prefer to have people inquiry privately, and then they provide pricing. It's difficult to know how much these prices fluctuate over time or whether they change depending on a consumer's inquiry. Be sure to do as much research as you can before making a purchase.

Risks

Microneedling is not suitable for everyone as it can exacerbate certain skin conditions such as active acne, eczema, and rosacea. It's also not recommended for individuals with a history of keloid scars or poor wound healing.

Just recently, I had a patient go to another aesthetic practitioner for microneedling. She didn't realize that we offer that service at our office. My team and I never brought it up to her as a good option because she has rosacea. Unfortunately, the other practitioner didn't screen her properly before moving ahead and performing the microneedling. Weeks after her treatment, she's still experiencing a rosacea flare and is back in contact with my office to help her manage it. It's much easier to avoid this kind of foreseeable issue than it is to treat it later.

This is one of the aesthetic treatments for which at-home devices have entered the market. Many patients wonder if they should get the treatment from a professional or buy the device and do it themselves at home. Some DIY devices may yield results, but professional devices can penetrate deeper into the skin, driving more-noticeable, long-lasting results. And with the use of any needle, it's important to be in a sterile environment in order to minimize the risk of infection. For this reason alone, microneedling at home is not recommended.

Platelet-rich plasma

PRP is a treatment that leverages the body's own healing processes to improve skin texture, tone, and overall appearance. It is derived from the patient's own blood, making it a natural and biocompatible treatment option with minimal risk of allergic reactions or side effects.

PRP is harvested by drawing a small amount of a patient's blood, typically from the arm. This blood is then placed in a centrifuge, a machine that spins the blood at high speed to separate its components based on their density. The centrifugation process separates the blood into three layers: red blood cells, plasma, and a concentrated layer of platelets known as platelet-rich plasma. The PRP layer, which is rich in growth factors and proteins, is then collected for use in treatment.

From there, the PRP is injected or applied topically to the target area, often combined with microneedling or laser treatments to enhance its absorption and effectiveness. PRP can be used on the face, neck, décolletage, scalp, or any other areas where rejuvenation is desired.

Platelet-rich plasma vs. Plasma-rich protein

These are terms that are often used interchangeably, but there are slight differences between them, albeit more in terminology and emphasis than in the fundamental substance or its application. Platelet-rich plasma and plasma-rich protein generally refer to the same substance derived from blood plasma that is rich in platelets and other proteins. The primary difference lies in the terminology and emphasis. Platelet-rich plasma focuses on the platelets' role, whereas plasma-rich protein can be seen as a broader term that includes the various proteins and growth factors present in the plasma. In practice, when clinicians refer to PRP in aesthetic or medical treatments, they almost always mean platelet-rich plasma, where the goal is to utilize the concentrated platelets and their associated growth factors for healing and rejuvenation.

How to use PRP

Direct injections: Direct injections allow for precise delivery of PRP to specific areas that require treatment, such as deep wrinkles, thinning hair, acne scars, surgical scars, uneven texture, or injured joints. I personally went through this procedure for my tennis elbow, and it was remarkable. I had tried physical therapy and all sorts of other modalities and nothing else was effective. However, PRP worked rather quickly.

There is also platelet-derived growth factor, which has made a lot of advances more recently. This is either used in conjunction with microneedling or injected into areas where there is volume loss, aging, or atrophy.

Microneedling with platelet-rich plasma: Often referred to as the "vampire facial," this involves applying PRP to the skin during or after microneedling. In layperson's terms, the practitioner extracts the patient's blood and smears it all over the patient's face. Because PRP is rich in growth factors, it enhances the healing process and improves overall results by further stimulating collagen production and tissue regeneration.

The first time I observed this treatment many years ago, I almost vomited. I was in the hallway talking to one of my partners after a treatment and realized the patient had blood smeared all over their face that they had to keep on their skin overnight! It was intense. And to think that we send people home like that to shock their family members!

One of my girlfriends called me the day after her treatment and said that her husband nearly fell off his chair when he saw her. He said, "Oh, my God! What did you do to your face? It looks like road rash, like you rubbed it in gravel." That said, it does work. She did a series of these treatments and came back for more. Her husband didn't object to any of it once he saw the results. In fact, she sent me a message from a beach in the US Virgin Islands saying, "He looked at me and said, 'Honey, your face and skin look so good. Did you get something else done? Your skin just looks so good.'" She looked as good on the outside as she felt on the inside.

That's the entire goal of this for us practitioners, isn't it? I find so much joy knowing that I played a small part in her ability to relax and enjoy her vacation with her husband, where she felt adored and beautiful.

Filler: In combination with other treatments such as dermal fillers, PRP can be used to enhance facial volume and contouring.

Hair restoration: PRP is an effective way to stimulate hair growth, whether a patient has androgenic alopecia (pattern baldness) or other hair thinning/loss. When injected into the scalp, or microneedling first and then PRP, this can stimulate dormant hair follicles, increase blood flow to the area, and thus promote new hair growth. It is often used in combination with other hair-restoration therapies.

Post-procedure healing: PRP is sometimes used after cosmetic or medical procedures to speed up the healing process and reduce inflammation. For example, it can be done after a laser treatment to accelerate tissue repair and minimize downtime. However, due to its relatively high cost, industry-produced post-procedure products are typically used instead. I also find that patients with sensitive skin do better with proprietary products, such as exosomes or post-procedure repair complexes, than with PRP.

Safety

You should never purchase PRP from another person, as each patient uses their own blood to make their own PRP. There have been incidents of unlicensed med spas having used pre-purchased PRP on patients and given them HIV. What a catastrophic mistake.

Even when your patients are using their own blood to make PRP, simply working with blood adds another layer of complication to your practice. It's essential to have a sterile environment and take the proper safety steps.

PRP isn't safe for everyone

As a practitioner, it's important to screen your patients for health issues and not provide services for those that present extra risk factors.

- **Cancer patients and survivors:** PRP is rich in growth factors that stimulate cell proliferation, tissue regeneration, and healing. Though this is beneficial in many contexts, for individuals with a history of cancer, there's a theoretical concern that these growth factors could potentially stimulate the growth of residual cancer cells or encourage the recurrence of cancer. There is only limited research specifically studying the long-term effects of PRP in cancer survivors. Due to this uncertainty, some healthcare practitioners exercise caution and may recommend against PRP for individuals with a history of cancer, particularly those with a recent history or who are in remission but still under close monitoring.

- **People with autoimmune disease:** PRP involves concentrating the body's own platelets and growth factors, which are then reintroduced into the body. In individuals with autoimmune disease, wherein the immune system mistakenly attacks healthy cells, there's a concern that the reintroduction of concentrated immune components might provoke an unwanted immune reaction. Further, PRP is designed to initiate an inflammatory response, which is part of the healing process. However, in people with autoimmune conditions, this could potentially worsen inflammation or flare-ups of the disease. Autoimmune conditions often involve chronic inflammation, and adding more inflammatory stimuli could aggravate symptoms.

These are important warnings to pay attention to when screening patients for new services. We have talked about capitalism without care elsewhere in this book, and it's so important to set these checks and balances for your practice.

I have a long-time patient who suffered from hereditary hair loss. One day, she came in for an appointment and told me that she was longing to try PRP. Mind you, she was already on a regimen of hair-loss treatment that's recommended by AAD, but she heard of the potential of PRP to grow hair more successfully than with other types of treatment. Unfortunately, she had a history of many skin cancers, having had a squamous-cell carcinoma three years prior and a basal-cell carcinoma one year prior. Although all were non-melanoma (according to most dermatology experts, melanoma precludes you from being a candidate for several years), one of the cancers was on her scalp, which increased the risk of doing PRP in that area. I counseled her and explained that she was not a good candidate for PRP and that undergoing that treatment, especially on her scalp, could be dangerous.

I saw her for a skin-cancer follow-up visit later that year and she confessed that she had found somewhere else in town that didn't mind that she'd had a recent history of skin cancer on her scalp and injected her with PRP. I was at a loss for words. How could a practitioner allow this for her? I decided that we should look up current guidelines and recommendations together as a refresher. We talked about why the guidelines exist and the risks of not following them. She cried and said that she knew better from her last meeting with me but was in denial about her situation. Her hair loss was a tremendous emotional burden, and she wanted a fix. After that talk, she realized that she couldn't do any more PRP treatments. She is one of my most faithful patients now, and she regrets having gone elsewhere in desperation.

PRP is growing in popularity, and I expect that to continue. Though PRP can improve skin quality and stimulate natural processes, currently, it is not a substitute for dermal fillers or surgical procedures when significant volume loss or skin laxity is present. The effectiveness of PRP can vary from patient to patient, depending on factors such as age, overall health, and the area being treated—and multiple sessions may be required to achieve the desired results.

As technology advances, PRP will only become even more effective. More precise and efficient centrifugation methods are being developed. These can lead to better separation of platelets and higher concentrations of growth factors, making PRP treatments more potent and effective. Improved protocols for PRP preparation can lead to greater consistency in PRP quality across different treatments. This could enhance treatment outcomes and allow for more reliable predictions of patient responses.

As our understanding of platelet biology deepens, scientists may identify which specific growth factors and bioactive molecules are most beneficial for different conditions. This knowledge could be used to tailor PRP preparations for specific treatments, such as skin rejuvenation, hair restoration, or even orthopedic applications. Future PRP technology might also allow for the customization of PRP formulations, optimizing them for individual patients based on their unique biological profile or specific treatment needs. This is an exciting area for aesthetics as well as general medicine—and I'm interested in seeing where research will take us.

Exosomes

More and more people are starting to talk about exosomes, especially as they compare with PRP.

Exosomes are small extracellular vesicles, typically ranging from 30 to 150 nm in size, that are secreted by nearly all types of cells. They contain a variety of bioactive molecules, including proteins, lipids, and nucleic acids such as mRNA and microRNA. These vesicles facilitate communication between cells by transferring their contents, thereby influencing various biological processes.

In regenerative medicine, exosomes are recognized for their ability to modulate inflammation, promote tissue repair, and enhance cellular communication. They play a key role in the body's natural healing processes. Exosomes used in therapy are often derived from stem cells, particularly mesenchymal stem cells, which are known for their regenerative capabilities. These stem-cell-derived exosomes are believed to carry powerful signals that stimulate healing and tissue regeneration.

Where do exosomes come from in aesthetics? Here's where things get a little weird. Exosomes can come from a variety of sources, but currently, the most well known and widely available line of exosomes is transforming growth factor beta, or TGFB. It originated from four liposuction patients whose tissues were mixed together and put through a complex process to screen for bacteria, viruses, and fungi before being dried into powder. The result is a product that has about a thousand different proteins that include the highest concentration of growth factors in the body. It is much more potent than PRP, and less inflammatory, making it a good option for those who have autoimmune issues. Exosomes can speed up the healing process of certain aesthetic treatments, such as lasers, by about two days.

Recently, I was on stage at a SkinMedica summit and sat next to Gail Naughton, PhD, the inventor of the TNS line of products. Her firsthand account of discovering exosomes in TNS Recovery Complex was riveting. First, it is important to note that human neonatal fibroblast source is the most pure and highest yield of growth factor available. This is the source for TNS, and since it is grown in hypoxic conditions (5 percent oxygen versus approximately 21 percent ambient oxygen), it is superior at differentiation as it is "pluripotent." This means the cell is capable of differentiating into any cell type within the body (except placenta). This term is usually used in embryonic-stem-cell biology jargon. I'll try not to get into the weeds too much here with the details around this, but in a nutshell, it's a game changer that TNS Recovery Complex has ingredients that contain pluripotent stem cells. In contrast, current competitors on the market contain differentiated cells, such as adipocytes (fat cells), which are an example of adult stem cells. Although these adult differentiated cells help with tissue repair, they are not as potent as a product with neonatal pluripotency. For example, if a fat cell is already a fat cell, it cannot become anything else. However, whenever a neonatal cell is pluripotent, it is able to become anything it needs to be, so the efficacy is much higher for wound care and skin repair/healing.

When Dr. Naughton was first examining their product in the 2000s, she thought that maybe there was an artifact in the slide preparation. She knew that growth factors were present, along with other proteins. However, since then, with improved electron microscope technology, we now know that the particles she was seeing were exosomes! The product was approved and went to market without anyone knowing that it had this benefit. In fact, there are over 1 trillion exosomes in every bottle of TNS Recovery Complex, which is the highest level of exosomes on the market today. That's a key reason why it is so effective at treating fine lines and wrinkles while improving skin tone and texture. For Dr. Naughton, it was a combination of good luck paired with hard work and brilliance.

When exosomes are combined with microneedling, the resulting treatment benefits from the strengths of both components. Exosomes can also be combined with PRP that is rich in growth factors that promote healing and tissue regeneration, with the exosomes adding an additional layer of communication and signaling, potentially enhancing the regenerative effects. Exosomes can amplify the effects of PRP by promoting more efficient and targeted cellular-repair processes. This combination can improve outcomes in treatments aimed at skin rejuvenation, hair restoration, and healing injuries.

The results of exosome treatments can vary based on individual factors such as a patient's age, overall health, and specific condition being treated. Some patients may see noticeable improvements after a single session, while others may require multiple treatments in order to achieve desired outcomes.

At our clinic, we have started applying the TNS Recovery Complex after lasers and microneedling—our own secret sauce for success.

Topical use vs. injections

At the time of this writing, exosomes have been approved for topical use only. The science is still so new that we don't have a full understanding of the potential risks and complications of injecting it. That means it's not just "off label" to inject exosomes; it's actually illegal.

You may have heard about clinics being raided after practitioners had used exosomes as injections. Some knew that what they were doing was illegal, but many didn't. One reason for this is how the product has been misrepresented to practitioners. I once had a disturbing conversation with a sales rep from a distributor who told me that practitioners aren't approved to use the product as an injection, but if someone wanted to use it that way, they could just mix it with saline instead of hyaluronic acid. If you were to do that, you could lose your license and maybe even go to jail. Using a product topically versus injecting it crosses an important legal boundary. Yes, people are doing it. But the FDA and DEA are cracking down, and it's not worth the risk. If you advertise that you do exosome injections that work miracles and regrow hair, don't be surprised when the authorities show up at your office.

Exosomes aren't safe for everyone

The science is still so new that we don't fully understand the implications. As with PRP, I wouldn't use exosomes on someone with cancer or even a history of cancer.

The future of regenerative medicine is expanding so rapidly. At a recent cosmetic meeting in California, a leading plastic surgeon spoke about how billionaire tech individuals are funding research in this arena. I can only imagine the growth we will see over the next 5 to 10 years and beyond.

As you just dip your toe into this arena or grow your practice to focus more on regenerative aesthetic medicine, make sure you stay up to date on current laws and only use certified products. Always check the sources of the exosomes so that you know that you're buying a reputable product. Doing so will help uphold the safety of your patients as well as the industry-wide reputation of these exciting new treatment options.

CHAPTER 13

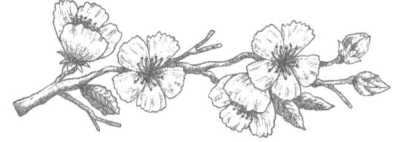

Putting It All Together

I had been working with patients for almost two decades before I really leaned into aesthetics. In 2020, I decided to try providing an advanced level of fillers at my practice. Allergan was offering a small amount of free product to practice with, but to qualify, I had to participate in a mandatory six-week online training given by Dr. de Maio to learn the new MD codes. Aesthetics trainings were offered regularly through a variety of sources, but until that point, they had always been a quick add-on or optional for me. As we all know, life has a way of getting busy. I'd always intended on going to more trainings, but I rarely traveled to any other states where the trainings were held. This time was different. I found my incentive and set aside time to devote to all six of the virtual training sessions, and the process ended up being a lightbulb moment for me. I had always loved the science behind aesthetic treatments, but now I could see that there was so much more to mastering it than I'd previously thought.

I was eager to try the injection strategies I'd learned and level up my skills. Although I had quite a bit of experience as an MD, as well as a decent amount of experience in the aesthetics space, I decided to provide some treatments to patients for free as I tried my hand at the new techniques I'd learned. I got a small quantity of products for free from Allergan to help me get more hands-on experience, but it wasn't much. I ended up giving away a lot of my time and definitely lost money that year. But the patients who got my free treatments loved their results. And they told their friends! Slowly but surely, I went on to gain a local following of loyal aesthetic patients.

I was wowed by how much the results meant to people. I was used to practicing general dermatology where my work fell squarely in the realm of physical health. Now I was doing work that was elective but had a transformative effect on the way people saw themselves. The sparkle came back into their eyes, they held their heads higher, and they left with a lightness in their spirit that wasn't there when they arrived. The treatments breathed new life into them from the inside. And in the same measure, I felt a part of myself awaken. That creative spark that had lain dormant for so long was reignited. After the difficult years of workplace burnout, COVID-19, and the drudgery that often comes in midlife, I remembered what it felt like to be fully alive.

I kept leaning into the aesthetics space to learn as much as I could. I went back to industry conferences I hadn't attended in more than five years and found even more to attend. I met interesting people I deeply admired. I learned about medical-grade skincare and became fascinated with the studies that scientifically proved how innovative new products had the power to change skin at a cellular level. Once again, I found myself dreaming of where my career might take me. I saw myself becoming a leader in the industry, speaking on stage at events to help others build their knowledge and regain their passion.

Back home in South Dakota, I brought my services out of "beta mode" and began charging a standard rate for them. Soon, my aesthetics practice was growing in triple digits year over year. I was invited to be on several aesthetics advisory boards, and my professional circle kept widening. In November 2023, I was selected to be one of 50 practitioners to attend a live training from Dr. de Maio where I learned even more about the nuances of injections. I hadn't thought much about my social media following, but it quickly grew from 50 followers to 100s, and I began sharing even more tips and tricks for skincare and aesthetic treatments.

After many years of maintaining the status quo, work felt new, fun, and exciting. I could tell that I was showing up differently for patients because I was living my passion. This created a totally different experience for them.

When it comes to aesthetic services, anyone can get people in the door, so the best way to differentiate yourself is to go beyond what people expect. You can't do this without being passionate about your work. In writing this book, my goal is to get practitioners excited to learn more about the industry and level up their skills. This is what worked for me.

I encourage you to explore different treatment modalities, strategies, and ways of working so that you can stay engaged. Figure out what interests you most and lean into that. Some practitioners have found success from carving out a specific niche in the industry. For example, if you're passionate about lip filler, don't be afraid to go all in on just that one service and become a master. But at the same time, don't feel like you have to narrow your expertise to develop a certain brand that doesn't feel authentic. There's no one right answer when it comes to going deep or broad. It's all about finding what works best for igniting your unique passion. You have to love what you do. After that, good outcomes will follow.

The real magic comes from combining treatment modalities

In this book, I've covered a wide variety of some of the most popular aesthetic treatments. All these modalities can make a difference as stand-alone treatments, depending on the patient's goals and preferences. But the real magic comes from combining these treatments in an individualized way to drive results that are greater than the sum of their parts. This is what separates the masters and artists from the technicians. When you step into the role of doing this kind of aesthetic strategy, not only is it more fulfilling and more interesting, but it also provides more value to patients.

To do this kind of work, you always start with a comprehensive consultation for new patients so you can understand their desired outcomes. From there, you create a recommended one-year plan, along with a separate plan for yearly maintenance.

Here are some of my favorite ways to combine aesthetic treatments to get results that go well beyond expectations:

Medical-grade skincare + aesthetic treatments in general: To make results go further, I always recommend pairing treatments with medical-grade skincare products. For example, if you want to use laser treatments to get rid of pigment, you need to pair it with a topical lightening agent so that the lasering continues to do the work after the treatment is over. My favorite is the LTN Complex in Even and Correct from SkinMedica. The same strategy is true when you use lasering for skin tightening or CoolSculpting to debulk tissue. If you pair these treatments with high-quality skincare products, such as SkinMedica's Firm and Tone or Revision's Bodifirm, the results will be more impressive and last longer.

Lasering + Botox + filler: Lasering is my go-to treatment for many patients, but the laser beam can't get into the deep crevices that some people have in their face. Botox helps get rid of those dynamic wrinkles that come from movement and prevents the crevices from becoming deeper so, over time and repeated use of Botox, those wrinkles are not as deep. Then, when you are lasered, the beam can reach the bottom of the crevice.

But this combo isn't just for fighting deep wrinkles. Botox doesn't help tighten the skin, so even if you keep it from moving as much, the skin is still getting bigger and starting to slowly sag. But when you combine lasering with Botox, they work synergistically and deliver exponentially better results than either treatment alone can. Skin becomes both smoother *and* tighter, which is typically the outcome that patients want.

From there, filler can help people look more youthful by adding volume in the right places. But it doesn't help tighten skin or get to the root cause of wrinkles. When you add filler after lasering and Botox, you have a higher-quality palette. You don't need as much filler as you otherwise would, and the results look even better.

BBL + Moxi: BBL lasers treat pigmentation, redness, and sun damage on the surface of the skin, whereas a Moxi laser (or similar) can go deeper to improve texture, wrinkles, and scars.

Combining these treatments targets both surface discoloration and deeper imperfections, leading to a more even and youthful complexion.

CoolSculpting + Kybella: When you use CoolSculpting to reduce fat under the chin, Kybella can be used afterward to further improve the appearance and texture of skin as well as decrease volume.

CoolSculpting or Kybella + RF: CoolSculpting and Kybella both reduce fat, whereas RF treatments firm and tighten the skin in the areas where fat has been reduced. This helps achieve both fat reduction and improved skin elasticity, resulting in a smoother and more contoured appearance.

Lasering + Ozempic: When you lose weight quickly, your skin can essentially become too big for your body. This causes exponential aging in the face. Patients who are dropping pounds quickly should consider monthly laser treatments on their face and neck.

Microneedling + RF: Microneedling promotes skin rejuvenation through collagen production, whereas radiofrequency uses heat to tighten the skin by stimulating deeper collagen fibers. This is such a great combination that a number of microneedling stamps have RF built into the heads. (Microneedling pens do not have RF, which is a key reason why they do not work as well.)

Microneedling + PRP or exosomes: Microneedling creates micro injuries in the skin in order to stimulate collagen production. When you combine it with PRP or exosomes, microneedling accelerates healing and boosts skin regeneration.

Do not underestimate the importance of making sure that foundational health and wellness elements are incorporated into all these treatments. This includes what I mentioned in earlier chapters, such as

Teach patients that they need to make the effort to do the little things between visits. This will create exponentially better long-term results and help them get the most out of their investment in professional aesthetic treatments

getting enough sleep, eating a nutritious diet, exercising, and wearing sunscreen and moisturizer every day. Our bodies are complicated systems, and every little bit of wellness support contributes to the big picture.

Another key point to understand is the importance of taking care of your skin over time, rather than waiting to correct it later. We apply this logic to other areas of life, but it's been slow to catch on in aesthetics. Think about it: would you wait until all your teeth fall out to go to the dentist? No. You brush them a couple times a day and get them cleaned two times a year so they don't fall out. Yes, you could let your teeth rot and then get dentures. But why would you put yourself through that invasive process when you could just take care of what you have?

The same logic should hold true for your skin. Teach patients that they need to make the effort to do the little things between visits. This will create exponentially better long-term results and help them get the most out of their investment in professional aesthetic treatments.

How to build your aesthetics practice

When you lean into your role as a master aesthetic practitioner, you want to be strategic about your career path. There are several different ways to look at this, but here are the strategies that have made the biggest difference for me over the years.

Be a lifelong learner

We all recognize that there are inconsistencies in state laws, training requirements, and the certifications needed to provide various aesthetic services. Instead of complaining about it, everyone should make an effort to learn as much as they can and proactively level up the community. We are all better together—so let's start acting like it!

As technology evolves and we continue to uncover new insights from scientific research, there will always be more to learn. We're going through a time of exponential change, and it takes work to keep up with it and stay informed! Go out of your way to attend conferences, connect with industry leaders you admire, and read new scientific studies. Every company you buy supplies and products from has a commercial-business-development representative, and their job is to educate you on how to get the most out of their offerings. Reach out to them! I have many of my reps' numbers saved in my phone, and I text them regularly with questions. You know what? Most of them text me right back with answers. I might be bugging them sometimes (such as when I was doing research for this book!), but it's their job to help answer their customers' questions. My secret weapon for knowledge is the medical-science liaison for these companies, and I am not shy to reach out to them for relevant studies. They have a ton of resources at their fingertips, so don't be afraid to ask.

Share your knowledge

As you level up your expertise, remember that knowledge is meant to be shared. Let me be clear: this is a call for practitioners to step up instead of opting out. We need to help form a community rather than foster an adversarial relationship.

Train your team members so that everyone in your practice can improve together. This is important for maintaining a synergistic relationship that's enjoyable. And it doesn't stop there. You should become a resource to people outside of your practice as well.

Some aesthetic practitioners seem to be born with the right frame of mind for building a community. Nicholas Howland, MD, and Trevor Larson, RN, both embody the attitude we all need to have when it comes to helping one another. Trevor is most well known for his expertise in lip injections, but he specializes in a range of treatments for the face and body. He does a great job of sharing his knowledge not only with other practitioners but with patients as well. He wants people to be well informed on the techniques and strategies he uses that drive such powerful outcomes.

Many of us don't realize how involved patients have become in the industry; they want to learn about aesthetics. And if their practitioner isn't producing any content, they will just get the information from someone else. In poking around social media, I've found that a number of my patients follow other dermatologists and aesthetics leaders who post all the time. When I realized this, it really encouraged me to lean into social media and share my knowledge.

Spend your time wisely

I interviewed a host of successful aesthetics leaders when I was writing this book, and the one thing everyone had in common was that they spend their time wisely.

To start, successful practitioners always make sure they spend enough time with patients to fully understand them and thus be able to address their needs. They don't halfway listen to patients with their hand on the doorknob. They do a full consultation on the first visit, and they give people their undivided attention from there on out. That makes all the difference in not only driving the best possible outcomes but also giving patients a positive experience. Jacqueline Calkin, MD, told me that she thinks of her practice as being the Nordstrom of dermatology because she wants to provide excellent patient satisfaction that goes beyond expectations. That starts and ends by listening.

The tricky thing here, though, is figuring out how to plan for this level of service and properly schedule it. Your time is your most valuable asset, and it can be difficult to find the right balance when it comes to providing thorough service and protecting this asset.

Some practitioners intentionally overbook themselves throughout the day, anticipating that there will be no-shows. This is a surefire way to plan for a chaotic day, but many practitioners prefer it over losing money from empty time slots on the calendar. Whenever possible, I recommend not intentionally overbooking and instead collecting deposits. You can manage this in different ways, depending on what your needs are. Personally, I like to get deposits from people who are signed up for services that take longer to provide, such as filler. If someone on my team is going to set aside an hour of our time to provide this type of treatment, we need to get compensated whether the person shows up or not.

I also make sure we charge patients whenever they want to come back in after an initial consultation and discuss treatment options in detail. I have the patient make a separate appointment with one of my PAs, for which we charge a reasonable fee. This helps protect our time and allows us to weed out the people who are window-shopping and using us as a resource to learn but aren't serious about moving forward with a treatment at our clinic.

Another important way to protect your time relates to training your team members. When you bring people on board, you need to make sure they spend enough time training and shadowing you. Craig Teller, MD, takes training very seriously. Whenever he hires someone new, he has an internal standard and doesn't let them practice alone for the first year. This takes a significant investment in terms of both his time and money. He's found that his colleagues end up so well trained after a year that other practitioners often try to poach them. To protect his investment, he has new hires sign two-year contracts. He also makes sure his practice is a great place to work so people want to stay and grow. Turnover can be costly in terms of time and money, so keeping a good team is of paramount importance.

Know when to say no

As a service practitioner, you should not automatically take every patient that walks through your door. Patients are interviewing you, and you are also interviewing them. It needs to be a mutually good fit or else there could be difficulty for both of you down the road. Knowing which patients to take and which to let go is one of the hardest things for a practitioner. And usually, people only get good at it after a decent amount of trial and error. That's because people can surprise you. The better you get at foreseeing the future, the better off you'll be.

After working with thousands of patients over the years, I've come to realize that some people are never happy. It doesn't matter the outcome or what their experience was like; they are nearly impossible to please. These people are not ideal candidates. If you can weed them out during the intake process, you should.

There are a few ways to spot these people. One way is by asking them what treatments they've had in the past, how they felt about the results, and why. If you notice a trend of negativity, especially any bad-mouthing about other aesthetic practitioners, you can likely expect that trend to continue if you decide to work with them.

A patient's viewpoint of pricing can make a difference in their perception of the experience as well. Those who are incredibly wealthy can have unrealistically high expectations for both the experience in the clinic as well as the outcome. Those who have very limited budgets can also be difficult to please because treatments are such a large investment that they expect to be blown away by the outcome. In reality, results are often subtle, and it takes multiple sessions or a combination of treatments over time to drive those jaw-dropping results.

I heard this comment from a colleague years ago regarding difficult-to-please patients, and it has resonated with me ever since: "It's much better to see that patient's back side once as they walk away from your clinic than it is to see their front side five times." Now, of course I want patients to be happy with their results, and if they end up needing a few more units of Botox here or there, it's no big deal. But when they have unrealistic expectations, that's when it becomes a time suck. The challenge is spotting these patients up front and letting them know that your practice isn't the right fit for them.

Another way I end up turning patients away is when they have a certain budget for treatments and it isn't high enough to drive a noticeable change. I've had patients come in and tell me they have $400 to spend and ask what they should do. This is always odd to me because it isn't the way people approach other services. You wouldn't go to your mechanic when your car is acting funny and tell them you have $400 to make the car better. Things cost what they cost. Yes, I could sell a bottle of filler or some Botox and stay within their budget, but if it isn't going to give them the outcome they want, what's the point? They aren't going to be happy in the end, and I won't gain a loyal patient. It's better to tell them to save up a little and come back when they have a larger budget that would allow us to perform the best possible treatments to meet their goals.

Lastly, we need to know when to say no to patients because they have had enough. Bartenders have this aspect as part of their job, as they need to recognize when a person has had enough to drink and should be cut off instead of overserving them. It might sound weird to say this, but the same holds true in aesthetics. People can become obsessed with beauty treatments. It doesn't matter how much they've had done—they always want more. Unfortunately, more is not always more. They might come through your door eager to pay you for treatments, but the best thing you can do is to stop enabling them. When you feel like someone is going too far and creating an unnatural look or electing to have work done that will make them look worse, don't be afraid to turn down their business.

Know when to say yes

I spoke with Nicolas Howland, MD, a successful plastic surgeon in Utah. He told me that his mother used to ask him what kind of surgery he performed that day: good plastic surgery or bad plastic surgery. But she wasn't referring to quality. She was talking about whether he performed surgery that truly helped someone, such as correcting a cleft lip, or surgery that contributed to the vanity of the world, such as a breast augmentation. That perspective never sat well with Dr. Howland, and it took him time to articulate why. Finally, he came to the realization that helping someone with a cleft lip in Guatemala boosted their confidence as much as doing a breast augmentation on another patient here in the states. Aesthetic changes are a highly personal journey, and it is not our place to judge the value or impact of their procedures. Dr. Howland has an interesting podcast in which he shares these kinds of stories and experiences to remove the stigma and/or shame often associated with the motivations behind plastic surgery. He's worked hard to foster an emotionally supportive community for patients, and I find that highly admirable.

It's impossible for us to know what it's like to live in someone else's body. Sometimes people get teased relentlessly as children because of an unusual anatomical feature and now that's the only thing they seen when they look in the mirror. What doesn't seem like a big deal to us is a huge issue to them that weighs down their self-esteem. Our job isn't to trivialize our patients' concerns or tell young adults to wait until they're older after having thought about it more. We need to keep our judgments out of the treatment room and listen to our patients reasonably. Elective treatments can be life-changing for people. Let's not be unreasonable gatekeepers.

Remember why you're here

Dolores, a 66-year-old patient of mine, came in recently on one of the days I dedicate to Medicare patients. I saw her for an annual skin check and we chatted about how to take care of dry skin. When I was wrapping up the visit, she said there was just one more thing she wanted to discuss. She told me that she had been doing research on social media and was learning all about the lines on her face. She'd determined that she had marionette lines and wondered what she could do to treat them.

Dolores is part of the generation that wasn't taught about prejuvenation because most of the treatments we have available today were either not invented yet or not widely available when she was younger. Throughout her life, she hadn't done much to take care of her skin.

When older patients come in and want to start focusing on aesthetics, it's tricky because most of the treatments are designed for people 65 and under. As I mentioned when I talked about new-patient consultations earlier in this book, "skin age" doesn't always align with a patient's actual age. If an older patient has younger-looking skin, it might still be possible to make some good progress with a few aesthetic treatments. But from my experience, the patients who come in when they're over 65 and want to start focusing on having more youthful skin are not in this category.

To make a noticeable difference for Dolores, it would take many treatments, which would turn into a significant investment in terms of time and money. Her best option, if she truly wanted to look younger, would be a lower facelift. This would tighten the skin significantly, reducing wrinkles, fine lines, and, specifically, her marionette lines. I'd known Dolores for a long time and was quite certain that this was not what she wanted to hear. Facelifts cost upwards of tens of thousands of dollars (or more), and surgery should not be taken lightly, especially for older folks.

I started out by validating Dolores as being a beautiful human being. I told her that she's a healthy 66-year-old and that people of that age tend to have wrinkles. I advised that she could sink a lot of money and time into aesthetic treatments that probably wouldn't do enough to make a substantial difference or she could spring for a facelift. Or, I told her, she could take that money and travel. She immediately said, "Yes, I think I'll do that instead!"

When you don't feel good about how you look on the outside, or it doesn't match how you feel on the inside, it can cause distress. If this distress is easily fixable through aesthetics, it can be a great solution.

It's important to be honest with patients, and sometimes this is most difficult when there isn't much we can do to help them.

When people come to us, they want to feel beautiful. It doesn't always take a treatment to do that. Sometimes it's enough to simply validate their feelings, remind them that everyone ages, and advise them to spend their time and money on things that would drive greater joy.

As you move forward in mastering your craft, never forget that the primary purpose of aesthetics isn't to make people look better; it's to make them feel better about themselves. The industry isn't usually considered to be part of the mental-health space, but the services we provide are absolutely engrained in boosting self-esteem and confidence. Yes, we should all evaluate ourselves solely based on what's on the inside, but oftentimes that just isn't reality. People with negative body image are two to three times more likely to experience depression than those with a positive body image.[88] Additionally, body-image concerns are associated with increased social anxiety and isolation.[89] How you feel about yourself on a daily basis matters. When you don't feel good about how you look on the outside, or it doesn't match how you feel on the inside, it can cause distress. If this distress is easily fixable through aesthetics, it can be a great solution.

As practitioners, the work we do can make a resoundingly positive impact in our patients' lives. At the same time, like the rest of the medical community, we need to observe the Hippocratic oath and "do no harm."

The industry has a responsibility to address concerns, not present them. It should always be patient driven. In other words, ask, "What concerns you?" If they don't bring it up themselves, don't just suggest something you think the patient should worry about.

We need to remember this as it becomes easier and easier to achieve—or at least get much closer to—whatever a patient's ideal beauty standards are. We can reshape jawlines, create the appearance of cheekbones, and make eyes look bigger and brighter. We can regrow hair, eliminate acne, and make wrinkles disappear. The results that people dreamed of years ago are now within reach. But we need to make sure this isn't a slippery slope of people never feeling like they are enough.

Practitioners should take a more active role in being part of the solution rather than part of the problem. We can help teach patients how to feel good about themselves and like themselves regardless of how they look.

When it comes to aging, let's remind ourselves that our skin isn't meant to continue looking like that of a newborn baby. We might not love the look of wrinkles, but they show all the smiles and laugher we've had over the years. They reveal a life well lived. Let's do our best to be grateful and embrace aging gracefully. Doing so will encourage our patients to do the same.

Quick Guide for Aesthetic Treatments, by Age

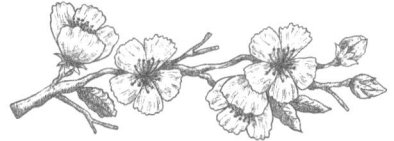

Here's my best advice for patients of all age groups.

Everyone

My first cardinal rule is to wear sunscreen on all sun-exposed skin every single day. This will be the least expensive thing you do for your skin and will have the highest yield. I have my favorite combo to wear that provides infrared protection and blue-light protection.

My second cardinal rule is to use a creamy moisturizer daily, ideally after you shower or bathe. Do these two things from a young age—or starting at any age, really—and you will be ahead of your peers!

Under 21

Although it's technically OK for anyone 18 or over to get aesthetic treatments, most services are intended for people 21 and up. It takes time for skin to reach maturity, and there's no need to provide skin treatments to younger, healthy skin. In fact, it can cause more harm than good. If a young person suffers from severe acne, that might be a different story, as the skin could benefit from certain treatments such as BBL, blue-light therapy, or another gentle light modality. But for most young people (or for that matter, anyone!), the best thing to do is to get into the habit of wearing moisturizer and sunscreen every single day.

One caveat to my reluctance in treating young people in this industry is when they have been extremely dissatisfied for a long time with a particular facial feature that is not going to change on its own. Examples of this could include having thin lips or a weak chin. If getting filler can make a big difference in self-esteem, I tend to think that the benefits of doing so outweigh the low risks of treatment—especially if it's a matter of getting the service sooner or later. Of course, this is a highly personal decision, and I don't believe in marketing these services to young people in an effort to create a need in the marketplace. When my daughter went to college, she got marketed to all the time by local clinics offering lip filler. Aesthetic practitioners who engage in this type of marketing are doing a disservice to society by targeting a highly impressionable demographic and potentially increasing their insecurities or making them feel worse about themselves.

21 to early 30s

People don't often think of this as a skincare treatment, but one of the easiest ways to safeguard against wrinkles is by wearing sunglasses. When you squint, the glabellar lines get deeper faster. All that squinting adds up over the years, and you can see it on people's faces. As if that weren't reason enough to wear sunglasses, there's also the fact that sunglasses help protect from developing macular degeneration.

In addition to wearing sunglasses religiously, for this age group, I advise patients to start leveling up their products to medical grade whenever possible. It can be pricy, so it's just a matter of how much people want to prioritize this as they earn a bit more money.

When it comes to treatments, most patients in this age group don't need a thing. That said, I do recommend lasers to patients if they had a lot of sun damage as a kid or have genetically loose skin and fine lines and wrinkles. We also do a substantial amount of lasering for these patients if they have had severe acne. If we're beginning to see fine lines in the forehead or around the eyes, early 30s could be the time to start thinking about Botox—and definitely sunglasses!

If patients are unhappy with the volume of their lips, this can also be a good time to experiment with a small amount of filler. This is also an age group that can use just a small amount of filler in the chin to see dramatic improvements in their profile and photos. There is a remarkable improvement in the fullness of the bottom lip when the chin is refined. (If patients are interested in lip filler, chin filler may actually be a better option!) Additionally, if patients are concerned with the appearance of submental fullness under the chin and are near their ideal weight, just one syringe of filler in the chin could reduce or eliminate that issue.

Mid 30s to early 40s

These are the prime years for remembering to use sunscreen on your neck and chest. An ounce of prevention can save a pound of damaged skin—and prevention is important for keeping your skin looking younger. This is a typical starting point for Botox, especially in and around the forehead, before permanent static lines are present. Lasering is also a great option for keeping the skin tight.

Late 30s is usually when we start to see some hollowing at the temples and midface, specifically on the cheeks. When you restore these areas with filler, you often don't need to fix the area under the eyes. It is so rewarding to use filler on the midface in this group since their skin quality is usually higher, they do not need as much filler, and a little goes a long way. Adding filler can provide dimension to patients who have a longer and more flat face. Augmenting the cheekbones can give a reflectivity of light that allows them to avoid makeup.

Remember that it's easier to maintain what you have than try to bring it back later after you've let it go, so antioxidant creams in the morning and restorative night treatments are high yield in this group—especially for people who live in more polluted areas.

Mid to late 40s

This can be a time to start becoming more conscious of the types of things that contribute to quicker aging. Whenever I find myself evaluating a patient and their age, my eye is invariably drawn to their neck and upper chest. How lax is the skin there? Is there a stark difference between the quality of the skin on their chest versus their face? If so, they might look much older than their actual age. Though I cannot stress enough the importance of protecting both of these areas, the dermis on the neck is virtually nonexistent compared with that of the face and therefore requires products that are specifically made to tighten the skin in that region. Don't forget that you can also use hyperdilute Botox in this area to decrease wrinkles and tighten the horizontal tech neck lines (horizontal wrinkles that appear on the neck due to prolonged periods of looking down at screens). Also, age spots on the chest can be reversed with cryotherapy (freezing) or laser. Whenever you find yourself tempted to lie in the sun and tan, remember that no one likes to look old when they wear a beautiful gown or bathing suit and you want to avoid developing crinkly skin between your breasts and on your upper chest.

Also, in your 40s, it is important to work diligently to decrease fine lines and wrinkles while protecting skin quality with lasers and medical-grade skincare. I know that I'm being repetitive, but wearing sunscreen daily on the face, neck, and chest is a must. Also, it is important to use laser treatments in order to maintain the integrity of the skin. In this age group, before the skin has too much laxity, I proceed with Botox before lasering. It helps to release dynamic movement and ensures that the laser can get down into the deeper areas of the smile lines.

In this age group, a lot of people notice how much they clench their jaw when they sleep. The most obvious repercussion here is that it can make teeth shift out of position or become cracked or chipped. When patients experience this, it's smart to see a dentist and look into getting a night guard to protect the teeth. On top of this, long-term clenching can cause increased wrinkling around the mouth, which is that pinched-up look that some people get. It makes it look as though they have a tremendous amount of stress in their life, and it truly decreases volume around the mouth. It also makes the jaw muscles get larger, which can noticeably change the shape of the face. Botox can be a huge help here when it comes to prevention. Start with 15 to 20 units per masseter. Another place to add up to an additional two units is the temporalis muscle (a muscle used for chewing).

Late 40s to 65

The best step forward here truly depends on a patient's skin age rather than their actual age. For patients who have older-looking skin, as well as those who are just dipping their toe into aesthetics, I recommend starting with a laser. Generally speaking, the older looking the skin is, the more aggressive you should go with the laser. If the patient has significant wrinkles and loose skin and they are open to total resurfacing, that's what will make the biggest difference right away. This is the erbium laser that is a ProFractional laser, and it is a power hitter for wrinkles. However, a lot of people these days don't like the 7- to 14-day downtime that comes with this option. If they want something less aggressive, you could recommend the Halo or Moxi. Just know that multiple treatments will likely be needed no matter which laser treatment they choose. Less-aggressive lasers typically turn into more appointments in order to yield the same outcomes.

Starting with a laser is important because it tightens the skin, which gives a better starting point for other treatments. (If you inject filler without tightening the skin first, it could end up looking droopy and requiring more filler.)

After a few laser sessions, I would opt to move forward with Botox. I would inject it full face and then have the patient come back in two weeks to see how it settles. Here's where the artistry really comes in. When the skin envelope is looser, Botox can fall a bit more than on tighter skin, and you might need to make adjustments. If more laser is needed to get down into where the wrinkles are deepest and are now exposed with Botox, then an additional session of laser could be beneficial.

From there, I usually recommend filler. As people age, they lose volume in their face. The muscles don't have as much to grab onto. We add filler to focus on vertical restoration, with the top priority usually being the temples. From there, we focus on the midface, adding filler to the cheeks. Often, once the midface has been restored, patients won't need much in the way of under-eye filler. Once that's stable, we can focus on the lower third of the face. If they have any jowl or pre-jowl groove, I add filler on the sides, then closer to the chin to bridge the jowl to the chin.

Over 65

Although most treatments are designated for people 65 and under, you can go by "skin age" rather than a patient's actual age. When patients have younger-looking skin, a laser, Botox, or filler can be a good option. For those with older-looking skin, a facelift might be the only option to make a real difference, especially to the neck. Many patients could benefit from a lower facelift, and I am very grateful that this option exists. I counsel patients to consider this option when it would be too costly to do repeated fillers and lasers. But of course, that comes with a hefty price tag as well, and risk.

It's great to have a few top-notch plastic surgeons you can recommend to your patients who want to go this route. Over the years, I've cultivated a strong network of practitioners I deeply trust, and I am so grateful for their skill and talent. I feel confident referring patients to them, and it's a huge weight off my shoulders to know that they will be in good hands. I recommend taking the time to research practitioners in your area, networking with them, and determining who could help care for your patients who want to go the surgical route.

Though I often can't in good conscience sell my older patients aesthetic services, that doesn't mean I don't have other advice for them. My top tip is to hydrate, hydrate, hydrate. If an older person comes into my clinic with properly hydrated skin, I'm shocked. It takes real effort and dedication to keep the skin hydrated as you age, but it's essential for skin health. And from an aesthetic perspective, hydrated skin looks younger. Refer back to chapter 6 and tell your patients to soak and seal within the first five minutes of getting out of the shower. For the hard-to-reach places, they should use Aquaphor in a spray bottle. Just make sure they apply it on a non-slip surface and have the ventilation on. Lotion can be slippery, and we don't want these patients falling down.

I also give them a handout of creams they can apply to their skin to help soften and even out the bumps that happen with age. These are often called "barnacles of wisdom" by the derm community, and their medical diagnosis is seborrheic keratosis. There are plenty of products on the market that can soften and thin these barnacles, such as CeraVe SA, Eucerin Roughness Relief Cream, and AmLactin.

For bruising, they can try a cream with arnica. My favorite drugstore brand for this is DerMend Moisturizing Bruise Formula, and my patients use it on their forearms to help with those areas affected by bruising with age.

Another nice recommendation can be Latisse—for growing not just thicker eyelashes but thicker eyebrows as well. Although it's off-label, Latisse can help with the thinning eyebrows that people often experience as they age. I tell patients to put one drop of Latisse into the bottle cap instead of putting a drop on each brush and use the brush to apply it to eyelashes before applying the leftover drop in the cap to their eyebrows. This conserves the product better so they won't need more of it in order to add their eyebrows to their beauty routine.

Quick Guide for Spotting Cancer

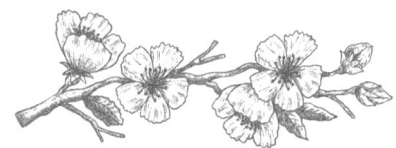

In the world of aesthetics, we look at skin all day every day. That's why practitioners are uniquely positioned to play a critical role in the early detection of skin cancer. By simply knowing what to look for when it comes to skin cancer, we can save lives.

I implore you to commit the details in this section to memory as much as you can and to keep coming back to this information whenever you need to reference it. You might even want to take a picture of these pages and save it to your phone! With a trained eye, you can absolutely identify suspicious features that warrant further medical evaluation. It's not a question of *if* you will spot skin cancer on a patient but *when*.

Over the years, I've spotted countless occurrences of skin cancer on my aesthetic patients. People look at their face every day and see fine lines and wrinkles, but they somehow fail to notice a suspicious little bump.

You must be prepared to be the person that will help them spot that little bump! Recognizing the signs of skin cancer early is crucial for effective treatment.

The three most common types of skin cancer are **basal-cell carcinoma**, **squamous-cell carcinoma**, and **melanoma**.

Here's how to spot each type of skin cancer:

1. Basal-cell carcinoma

- **Appearance:** Basal-cell carcinoma often appears as a small, pearly, pink, or shiny bump on the skin. It may also look like a flat, flesh-colored, or brown scar-like or rash lesion.
- **Location:** It is commonly found on sun-exposed areas such as the face, ears, neck, scalp, shoulders, and back.
- **Growth:** It grows slowly and may bleed or develop a crust. If untreated, it can cause significant damage to surrounding tissue but rarely spreads to other parts of the body.

2. Squamous-cell carcinoma

- **Appearance:** Squamous-cell carcinoma may appear as a firm, red nodule or a flat lesion with a scaly, crusted surface. It can also look like a rough, scaly patch that may bleed or form a sore.
- **Location:** It commonly appears on sun-exposed areas such as the face, ears, neck, hands, and arms.
- **Growth:** It tends to grow more rapidly than basal-cell carcinoma and can become invasive, potentially spreading to other parts of the body if left untreated.

3. Melanoma

- **Appearance:** Melanoma can develop in an existing mole or appear as a new, unusual growth. Use the following "ABCDE" guideline to help identify potential melanomas:
    - **A**symmetry: One half of the mole doesn't match the other.
    - **B**order: The edges are irregular, ragged, notched, or blurred.
    - **C**olor: The color is uneven, with shades of brown, black, tan, red, white, or blue.
    - **D**iameter: Melanomas are usually larger than 6 mm (about the size of a pencil eraser) but can be smaller.
    - **E**volving: The mole changes in size, shape, or color or begins to itch or bleed.

- **Location**: It can appear anywhere on the body, including areas not exposed to the sun, such as the soles of the feet, palms, or under the nails.
- **Growth**: Melanoma can spread quickly to other parts of the body, making early detection and treatment critical.

Other warning signs

- **Sores that don't heal**: A sore that doesn't heal or keeps coming back could be a sign of skin cancer.
- **Changes in an existing mole**: Any changes in the color, size, or texture of a mole should be checked.
- **New growths**: Any new growths, especially those that look different from other moles or spots on your body.
- **Redness or swelling**: beyond the border of a mole.
- **Itching or tenderness**: Persistent itching, tenderness, or pain in a specific area.

When to speak up

One in five Americans will get skin cancer at some point in their lifetime.[90] Anyone can get skin cancer, regardless of age or skin color. If you see something that could be suspicious, ask your patient about it. Ask if they've had a skin check recently by a dermatologist. Inquire as to whether they've noticed any changes with marks, bumps, or moles. Make a note in your file if you see something suspicious, or even ask the patient to take a photo of it that day to help monitor if it changes over time. If you take good notes or have a photo to reference, it's quite possible that you'll see a patient a few times and be able to notice changes yourself.

You might even want to get pamphlets or brochures that help your patients identify the signs of skin cancer to have on hand at your office.

To be clear, as an aesthetic practitioner, to make a real difference in someone's life, you don't have to be the person that diagnoses the skin cancer. You just need to point out what you see and make sure your patient knows how serious it is that they get checked out by a dermatologist. Tell your patients that regular skin checks are important, especially for those with a history of excessive sun exposure or a family history of skin cancer.

Many insurance plans cover annual skin checks, so it's usually not cost prohibitive. For those without this kind of insurance, many health systems offer free screenings in May, which is Skin Cancer Awareness Month. You can find more information on the AAD website. Just search for "AAD free skin cancer check."

As aesthetics professionals, we are a vital line of defense in spotting skin cancer early, when it is most treatable. At the end of the day, helping a person look and feel their best is rewarding, but nothing compares to adding years to their life.

Acknowledgments

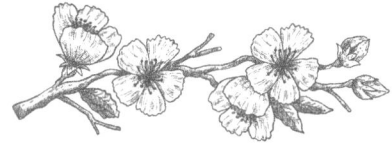

I would like to first thank my husband, who supports me to no end. We are so lucky we found each other. I am grateful to have your rock-solid support.

To my three daughters, who had my heart from the moment I first laid eyes on them. Without you, I would not have been able to take on this endeavor. From jumping in and helping with research to family summer evenings going over nutrition and current guidelines, our entire family time has essentially been the summer of "my book." You are my core, and I adore you all.

To my parents, who told me I could do anything. You said it so often that I believed it—and it became a given. Dad, you are the epitome of support to this day. Mom would have loved this. I know she is smiling from above.

To my sister, who always offers to pitch in, do recon on social media, find me stellar outfits, listen to my stories about interviews, and help promote me.

To all the interviewees who spent countless hours on Zoom with me, thank you. I learned so much, and I am inspired and truly challenged to be as outstanding as each and every one of you.

To my friends and family who supported this idea from the outset, I am so grateful for all of you. Only positive comments, and such encouragement. For those of you who offered and did help with ideas and feedback, thank you.

To all my professors and mentors along the way, you helped to shape me. I couldn't have accomplished college, medical school, and residency without you. To my partners and admin who have supported me during this process, thank you.

Finally, to Amelia Forczak, who was there each step of the way during this year-long journey. Your guidance, direction, feedback, and encouragement helped me when this felt insurmountable. Thank you to the whole Pithy Wordsmithery team, an indispensable resource for writers everywhere who just want to get started.

About the Author

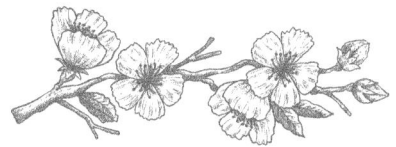

Lycia Thornburg, MD, FAAD, is a board-certified dermatologist who is passionate about the health of her patients' skin and known for her dedication to both cutting-edge research and compassionate patient care. One of her central focuses is educating patients about protecting their skin, thereby preventing and lessening dermatologic diseases.

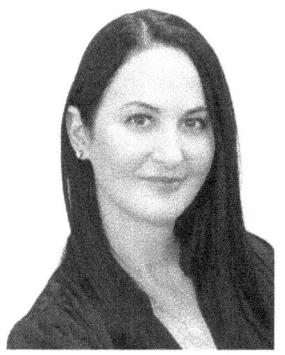

Originally from Waukesha, Wisconsin, her journey into medicine began with a Bachelor of Science from the University of Wyoming. She went on to earn her medical degree from the Medical College of Wisconsin, followed by dermatology residency at the University of Iowa Hospitals and Clinics, where she honed her expertise in skin health.

She has been practicing dermatology in Rapid City, South Dakota, since 2003 and has become renowned for her wide-ranging expertise in general, laser, and aesthetic dermatology. Her clinical work reflects a deep commitment to the intersection of aesthetics and medical dermatology.

She serves on several national advisory boards for skincare, Botox, and filler. Dr. Thornburg recently presented on stage for SkinMedica as a national expert on growth factors.

As a respected voice in the field, she serves as a national media expert for AAD and appears on a monthly television segment educating the public on national awareness issues in dermatology. Representing dermatologists about skin health and care, her publications include articles in *Better Homes and Gardens, New Beauty, InStyle,* and on Byrdie.com.

Beyond her professional accolades, Dr. Thornburg is deeply invested in public health. In 2007, she founded the charity Made for Shade, a pioneering initiative aimed at protecting children from the harmful effects of sun exposure while promoting healthy outdoor activities. Each year, she and Made for Shade host an annual food- and wine-tasting event to raise awareness and funds to prevent skin cancer in her region. This event has grown each year and has become an example for other regions on how to protect children from harmful UV rays.

Dr. Thornburg's contributions extend to dermatological research, where she collaborates on groundbreaking studies evaluating cancer biomarkers through an inter-departmental research collaborative effort in her clinic.

Her patient-care philosophy is as much about emotional well-being as it is about physical health. Inspired by Maya Angelou's words—"People will forget what you said, people will forget what you did, but people will never forget how you made them feel"—she brings empathy and understanding to each patient interaction, creating a holistic approach that sets her apart in the world of dermatology. Her goal is to help patients feel the same way on the outside as they do on the inside.

Outside her practice, Dr. Thornburg enjoys spending time with her husband and family, especially supporting her daughters in their endeavors. They share a love for travel and adventure and enjoy skiing, going to the beach, and gardening (some more than others!). They have three dogs that keep them entertained as only doodles can do.

Endnotes

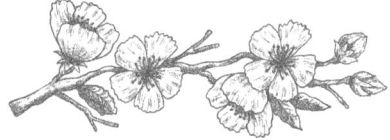

1 Fortune Business Insights. Cosmetics Market Size, Share & Industry Analysis, by Category (Hair Care, Skin Care, Makeup, and Others), by Gender (Men and Women), by Distribution Channel (Specialty Stores, Hypermarkets/Supermarkets, Online Channels, and Others), and Regional Forecasts, 2024–2032. Last Updated July 29, 2024, accessed August 17, 2024, https://www.fortunebusinessinsights.com/cosmetics-market-102614.

2 neuromodulator: something (as a polypeptide) that potentiates or inhibits the transmission of a nerve impulse but is not the actual means of transmission itself (Merriam-Webster online), https://www.merriam-webster.com/medical/neuromodulator.

3 "Hilary Wilson on… Mirrors in Ancient Egypt," The Past, August 7, 2023, https://the-past.com/feature/hilary-wilson-on-mirrors-in-ancient-egypt/.

4 Ann Liljas, "Old age in ancient Egypt," UCL, March 2, 2015, https://blogs.ucl.ac.uk/researchers-in-museums/2015/03/02/old-age-in-ancient-egypt/#:~:text=However%20we%20do%20know%20that,prescriptions%20for%20face%20and%20skin.

5 Judith Illes, "Ancient Egyptian Eye Makeup," Tour Egypt, August 9, 2011, https://www.touregypt.net/egypt-info/magazine-mag09012000-mag4.htm.

6 Laura Gariepy, "Women and Credit: A Look at the History," *U.S. News and World Report*, March 22, 2024, https://money.usnews.com/credit-cards/articles/women-and-credit-a-look-at-the-history#:~:text=This%20year%20marks%20the%2050th,take%20ownership%20of%20their%20lives.

7 "New report: Physically attractive people earn 15% more than plainer colleagues," IZA World of Labor, June 29, 2015, accessed August 17, 2024, https://wol.iza.org/press-releases/does-it-pay-to-be-beautiful.

8 Cathy Cassata, "TikTok Is the Main Source of Health Information for a Third of Gen Z, Survey Finds," Healthline, July 8, 2024, accessed August 17, 2024, https://www.healthline.com/health-news/tiktok-main-source-health-information-gen-z.

9 Sam Meredith, "Facebook-Cambridge Analytica: A timeline of the data hijacking scandal," CNBC, April 10, 2018, https://www.cnbc.com/2018/04/10/facebook-cambridge-analytica-a-timeline-of-the-data-hijacking-scandal.html.

10 Nicholas Confessore, "Cambridge Analytica and Facebook: The Scandal and the Fallout So Far," *The New York Times*, April 4, 2018, https://www.nytimes.com/2018/04/04/us/politics/cambridge-analytica-scandal-fallout.html.

11 Amir Reza Ashraf et al., "Safety and Risk Assessment of No-Prescription Online Semaglutide Purchases," JAMA Network, August 2, 2024, https://jamanetwork.com/journals/jamanetworkopen/fullarticle/2821882.

12 nutraceuticala: foodstuff (such as a fortified food or dietary supplement) that provides health benefits in addition to its basic nutritional value (Merriam-Webster online), https://www.merriam-webster.com/dictionary/nutraceutical.

13   "Why take vitamin and mineral supplements?" Mayo Clinic, August 23, 2022, accessed July 14, 2024, https://www.mayoclinichealthsystem.org/hometown-health/speaking-of-health/why-take-vitamin-and-mineral-supplements#:~:text=Select%20a%20vitamin%20that%20provides,Ask%20the%20experts.

14   "Vitamins and Minerals: What You Should Know About Essential Nutrients," Mayo Clinic, accessed July 14, 2024, https://www.mayoclinic.org/documents/mc5129-0709-sp-rpt-pdf/doc-20079085.

15   Rabail Javed et al., "Levels of 25-OH Vitamin D in Healthy Asymptomatic Adults: Pilot Study," Park J Med Res., Vol. 51, No. 3, 2012, https://applications.emro.who.int/imemrf/Pak_J_Med_Res/Pak_J_Med_Res_2012_51_3_82_86.pdf.

16   Ibid.

17   Heike A Bischoff-Ferrari et al., "Estimation of optimal serum concentrations of 25-hydroxyvitamin D for multiple health outcomes2," *The American Journal of Clinical Nutrition,* Volume 84, Issue 1, 2006, 18–28, ISSN 0002-9165, https://doi.org/10.1093/ajcn/84.1.18.

18   Ghada El-Hajj Fuleihan et al., "Serum 25-Hydroxyvitamin D Levels: Variability, Knowledge Gaps, and the Concept of a Desirable Range," *Journal of Bone and Mineral Research,* Volume 30, Issue 7, July 1, 2015, 1119–1133, https://doi.org/10.1002/jbmr.2536.

19   Bess Dawson-Hughes et al., "Estimates of optimal vitamin D status," *Osteoporos Int* 16, 2005, 713–716, https://doi.org/10.1007/s00198-005-1867-7.

20   Matthias Wacker and Michael F Holick, "Sunlight and Vitamin D: A global perspective for health," *Dermato-endocrinology,* vol. 5,1, 2013, 51–108, doi:10.4161/derm.24494.

21   Mohana Chakkera et al., "The Efficacy of Vitamin D Supplementation in Patients With Alzheimer's Disease in Preventing Cognitive Decline: A Systematic Review," *National Library of Medicine,* November 20, 2022, https://pubmed.ncbi.nlm.nih.gov/36569670/.

22   Antonia Pignolo et al., "Vitamin D and Parkinson's Disease," Mar 14, 2022;14(6):1220. doi: 10.3390/nu14061220. PMID: 35334877; PMCID: PMC8953648.

23   Sneha Baxi Srivastava, "Vitamin D: Do We Need More Than Sunshine?" *American Journal of Lifestyle Medicine,* vol. 15,4, 397–401, April 3, 2021, doi:10.1177/15598276211005689.

24   Katherine Zeratsky, "What is vitamin D toxicity? Should I be worried about taking supplements?" Mayo Clinic, accessed July 14, 2024, https://www.mayoclinic.org/healthy-lifestyle/nutrition-and-healthy-eating/expert-answers/vitamin-d-toxicity/faq-20058108#:~:text=The%20main%20consequence%20of%20vitamin,the%20formation%20of%20calcium%20stones.Nutrition.

25   Andrew C. Chen et al., "A phase 3 randomized trial of nicotinamide for skin cancer chemoprevention," *The New England Journal of Medicine,* October 22, 2015, https://www.nejm.org/doi/full/10.1056/NEJMoa1506197.

26   Vitamin B3 (Niacin), Mount Sinai website, https://www.mountsinai.org/health-library/supplement/vitamin-b3-niacin#:~:text=Anticoagulants%20(blood%20thinners)%3A%20Niacin,risk%20of%20low%20blood%20pressure.

27   Farid Mallat et al., "Botulinum Toxins and Zinc: From Theory to Practice-A Systematic Review," National Library of Medicine, June 20, 2023, https://pubmed.ncbi.nlm.nih.gov/37335837/.

28   Anne Guertler, "Exploring the potential of omega-3 fatty acids in acne patients: A prospective intervention study," Wiley Online Library, July 10, 2024, https://onlinelibrary.wiley.com/doi/10.1111/jocd.16434.

29   Szu-Yu Pu et al., "Effects of Oral Collagen for Skin Anti-Aging: A Systematic Review and Meta-Analysis," *Nutrients*, vol. 15,9, 2080, April 26, 2023, doi:10.3390/nu15092080.

30   free radical: an especially reactive atom or group of atoms that has one or more unpaired electrons, especially one that is produced in the body by natural biological processes or introduced from an outside source (such as tobacco smoke, toxins, or pollutants) and that can damage cells, proteins, and DNA by altering their chemical structure (Merriam-Webster online), https://www.merriam-webster.com/dictionary/free%20radicals.

31   Robert Shmerling, "Coffee May Help Your Skin Stay Healthy," Harvard Health Publishing, November 2, 2018, https://www.health.harvard.edu/blog/coffee-may-help-your-skin-stay-healthy-2018110215295.

32   Kurek-Górecka et al., "Bee Products in Dermatology and Skin Care," *Molecules*, January 28, 2020, https://www.ncbi.nlm.nih.gov/pmc/articles/PMC7036894/pdf/molecules-25-00556.pdf.

33   Zoe Diana Draelos, "Sugar Sag: What Is Skin Glycation and How Do You Combat It?" *J Drugs Dermatol*, 2024;23:4(Suppl 1):s5-10, https://jddonline.com/articles/individual-article-sugar-sag-what-is-skin-glycation-and-how-do-you-combat-it-S1545961624SSF378083s5X.

34   "What is Skin Cancer?" Illinois Department of Public Health. Skin Cancer, accessed July 6, 2024, https://dph.illinois.gov/topics-services/diseases-and-conditions/diseases-a-z-list/skin-cancer.html.

35   "Skin Cancer Facts & Statistics," Skin Cancer Foundation, accessed July 6, 2024, https://www.skincancer.org/skin-cancer-information/skin-cancer-facts/.

36   Ultraviolet (UV) Radiation Tanning Equipment , EPA, accessed July, 14, 2024, https://www.epa.gov/radtown/ultraviolet-uv-radiation-tanning-equipment.

37   Candance Flores, "Light and Infrared Radiation," Environment, Health, & Safety, June 7, 2018, https://ehs.lbl.gov/service/radiation-protection/non-ionizing-radiation/.

38   T. Passeron et al., "Photoprotection according to skin phototype and dermatoses: practical recommendations from an expert panel," National Library of Medicine, May 4, 2021, 1460–1469, https://pmc.ncbi.nlm.nih.gov/articles/PMC8252523/#:~:text=Tinted%20sunscreens%20containing%20pigments%2C%20particularly,for%20intermediate%20and%20dark%20skin.

39   Cosmetic Products Regulation, Annex VI - Allowed UV Filters, ECHA, accessed July 14, 2024, https://echa.europa.eu/cosmetics-uv-filters.

40   "FDA in Brief: FDA announces results from second sunscreen absorption study," FDA, accessed July 14, 2024, https://www.fda.gov/news-events/fda-brief/fda-brief-fda-announces-results-second-sunscreen-absorption-study#:~:text=The%20publication%20results%20show%20that,levels%20of%20the%20active%20ingredient.

41 Skin Cancer: Facts and Stats, Dartmouth Geisel School of Medicine, accessed July 6, 2024, https://geiselmed.dartmouth.edu/students/student-wellness-resources/sun-safety-and-skin-cancer-prevention/skin-cancer-facts-and-stats.

42 Fiona McNeill, "Analysis: Dying for makeup – Lead cosmetic poisoned 18th-century European socialites in search of whiter skin," McMaster University, February 28, 2022, https://brighterworld.mcmaster.ca/articles/analysis-dying-for-makeup-lead-cosmetics-poisoned-18th-century-european-socialites-in-search-of-whiter-skin/.

43 Neonatal fibroblast tissue is a cell line derived from the foreskin of a newborn that can be used for a variety of research purposes(Google), https://www.google.com/search?q=neonatal+fibroblast+tissue&num=10&newwindow=1&sca_esv=d8dc71a00e7da157&rlz=1C1CHBF_enUS879US879&ei=9HgnZ--aLbzUp84PxKS9gQI&ved=0ahUKEwjv5JHroMCJAxU86skDHURSLyAQ4dUDCBA&uact=5&oq=neonatal+fibroblast+tissue&gs_lp=Egxnd3Mtd2l6LXNlcnAiGm5lb25hdGFsIGZpY-nJvYmxhc3QgdGlzc3VlMgUQIRigATIFECEYoAEyBRAhGKABMgUQIRigATIFECEYnwUyBRAhGJ8FSIcDUABYAHAAeAGQAQCYAXegAXeqAQMwLjG4AQPIAQD4AQL4AQGYAgGgApMBmAMAkgcDMC4xoAeXBg&sclient=gws-wiz-serp; mesenchyme: loosely organized undifferentiated mostly mesodermal cells that give rise to such structures as connective tissues, blood, lymphatics, bone, and cartilage (Merriam-Webster online), https://www.merriam-webster.com/dictionary/mesenchyme.

44 Kuniko Kadoya et al., "Upregulation of Extracellular Matrix Genes Corroborates Clinical Efficacy of Human Fibroblast-Derived Growth Factors in Skin Rejuvenation," National Library of Medicine, December 1, 2017, 1190–1196, https://pubmed.ncbi.nlm.nih.gov/29240854/.

45 Zoe Diana Draelos et al., "Clinical Benefits of Circadian-based Antioxidant Protection and Repair," National Library of Medicine, December 1, 2020, https://pubmed.ncbi.nlm.nih.gov/33346522/.

46 Lauryn Reid et al., "Long-Term Efficacy and Tolerability of a Daily Serum for Rejuvenation and Prejuvenation of Facial Skin," *Journal of Drugs in Dermatology*, August 22, 2023, 917–924, https://jddonline.com/articles/long-term-efficacy-and-tolerability-of-a-daily-serum-for-rejuvenation-and-prejuvenation-of-facial-skin-S1545961623P0917X/.

47 Andrew C. Chen et al., "A Phase 3 Randomized Trial of Nicotinamide for Skin Cancer Chemoprevention," *The New England Journal of Medicine*, October 22, 2015, https://www.nejm.org/doi/full/10.1056/NEJMoa1506197.

48 Ibid.

49 Ryan C. Kelm et al., "Effective Lightening Of Facial Melasma During The Summer With A Dual Regimen: A Prospective, Open-Label, Evaluator-Blinded Study," National Institutes of Health, December 19, 2020, 3251–3257, https://pubmed.ncbi.nlm.nih.gov/33058522/.

50 ATP: adenosine triphosphate (ATP), energy-carrying molecule found in the cells of all living things. ATP captures chemical energy obtained from the breakdown of food molecules and releases it to fuel other cellular processes (Britannica online), https://www.britannica.com/science/adenosine-triphosphate.

51 Elizabeth T. Makino et al., "Clinical Efficacy of a Novel Two-Part Skincare System on Pollution-Induced Skin Damage," *Journal of Drugs in Dermatology,* September 2018, 975–981 https://jddonline.com/articles/clinical-efficacy-of-a-novel-two-part-skincare-system-on-pollution-induced-skin-damage-S1545961618P0975X/.

52 Morgann B Young et al., "A Rejuvenating treatment targeting 'tech neck' lines and wrinkles in Chinese women: A prospective, open-label, single-center study," National Library of Medicine, November 14, 2022, 226–235, https://pubmed.ncbi.nlm.nih.gov/36374589/.

53 Elizabeth T. Makino, et al., "Efficacy and Tolerability of a Novel Topical Treatment for Neck: A Randomized, Double-blind, Regimen-Controlled Study." *Journal of Drugs in Dermatology,* 2021, 184–191, https://jddonline.com/articles/efficacy-and-tolerability-of-a-novel-topical-treatment-for-neck-a-randomized-double-blind-regimen-co-S1545961621P0184X.

54 Sabrina G. Fabi et al., "Optimizing Facial Rejuvenation with a Combination of a Novel Topical Serum and Injectable Procedure to Increase Patient Outcomes and Satisfaction," *Journal of Clinical Aesthetic Dermatology,* 2017, 14–18, https://jcadonline.com/december-2017-optimizing-facial-rejuvenation/.

55 Ali Rajabi-Estarabadi et al., "Effectiveness and tolerance of multicorrective topical treatment for infraorbital dark circles and puffiness," National Library of Medicine, December 19, 2023, 486–495, https://pubmed.ncbi.nlm.nih.gov/38112168/.

56 "NASA Research Illuminates Medical Uses of Light," NASA, May 19, 2022, https://spinoff.nasa.gov/NASA-Research-Illuminates-Medical-Uses-of-Light.

57 chromophore: a chemical group (such as an azo group) that absorbs light at a specific frequency and so imparts color to a molecule (Merriam-Webster online), https://www.merriam-webster.com/dictionary/chromophore.

58 stratum corneum: the outermost layer of the epidermis that consists of keratin-rich corneocytes connected by desmosomes and embedded in a matrix of lipids (such as ceramides and cholesterol) arranged in bilayers and that regulates skin permeability, maintains hydration, provides structural integrity, and acts as a protective barrier (as against UV radiation, pathogens, and toxins) (Merriam-Webster online), https://www.merriam-webster.com/dictionary/stratum%20corneum.

59 port-wine stain: a reddish-purple superficial hemangioma of the skin commonly occurring as a birthmark (Merriam-Webster online), https://www.merriam-webster.com/dictionary/port-wine%20stains.

60 exosome: a tiny sac-like structure that is formed inside a cell and contains some of the cell's proteins, DNA, and RNA. Exosomes get released into the blood by many types of cells, including cancer cells, and travel through the blood to other parts of the body. (cancer.gov), https://www.cancer.gov/publications/dictionaries/cancer-terms/def/exosome.

61 Anne Kingston, "What you need to know about Botox from the Vancouver couple who pioneered it," Macleans, June 3, 2014, accessed July 26, 2024, https://macleans.ca/society/health/meet-the-vancouver-couple-who-pioneered-botox/.

62 Ibid.

63 Zachary Crockett, "The economics of Costco rotisserie chicken," The Hustle, updated June 24, 2024, https://thehustle.co/the-economics-of-costco-rotisserie-chicken.

64   temporalis: a large muscle in the temporal fossa that serves to raise the lower jaw and is composed of fibers that arise from the surface of the temporal fossa and converge to an aponeurosis which contracts into a thick flat tendon inserted into the coronoid process of the mandible (Merriam-Webster online), https://www.merriam-webster.com/medical/temporalis.

65   LJ Charleston, "The story of Gladys Deacon: The 1920s socialite who became a recluse and died in a mental hospital," news.com.au, August 11, 2019, https://www.news.com.au/lifestyle/real-life/true-stories/the-story-of-gladys-deacon-the-1920s-socialite-who-became-a-recluse-and-died-in-a-mental-hospital/news-story/c94037af12d6ec5d9b0ce6bce5526d6e.

66   Theda C. Kontis and Alexander Rivkin, "The History of Injectable Facial Fillers," 2009, https://westsideaesthetics.com/wp-content/uploads/2023/04/history-injectable-fillers-2009.pdf.

67   Christopher K. Hee et al., "Rheological Properties and In Vivo Performance Characteristics of Soft Tissue Fillers," National Library of Medicine, S373–S381, https://pubmed.ncbi.nlm.nih.gov/26618467/.

68   aseptic technique: a procedure that healthcare practitioners use to prevent the spread of germs that cause infection. Placing barriers, using sterile equipment and following strict guidelines help create an environment free of germs that can make you sick (Cleveland Clinic website), https://my.clevelandclinic.org/health/treatments/aseptic-technique.

69   granuloma: a mass or nodule of chronically inflamed tissue with granulations that is usually associated with an infective process (Merriam-Webster online), https://www.merriam-webster.com/dictionary/granuloma.

70   Steven Dayan, MD, *Subliminally Exposed* (Megan James Publishing 2013), 57.

71   Dr. Koenraad De Boulle and Dr. Izolda Heydenrych, "Patient factors influencing dermal filler complications: prevention, assessment, and treatment," *Dovepress*, 205–214, https://doi.org/10.2147/CCID.S80446.

72   necrotic: affected with, characterized by, or producing death of a usually localized area of living tissue (Merriam-Webster online), https://www.merriam-webster.com/dictionary/necrotic.

73   Derek H. Jones et al., "Preventing and Treating Adverse Events of Injectable Fillers: Evidence-Based Recommendations From the American Society for Dermatologic Surgery Multidisciplinary Task Force," *Dermatologic Surgery*, February 2021, 214–226, https://doi.org/10.1097/DSS.0000000000002921.

74   Matthew Halverson, "Sir Mix-a-Lot Reflects on 'Baby Got Back,' 20 Years Later," *Seattle Met*, April 25, 2012, https://www.seattlemet.com/news-and-city-life/2012/04/sir-mix-a-lot-reflects-on-baby-got-back-20-years-later-may-2012.

75   Anne Ewbank, "Looking Like a Flapper Meant a Diet of Celery and Cigarettes," *Atlas Obscura*, April 20, 2018, https://www.atlasobscura.com/articles/1920s-food-flapper-diet.

76   Lázaro Cárdenas-Camarena et al., "Strategies for Reducing Fatal Complications in Liposuction," National Library of Medicine, October 25, 2017, https://www.ncbi.nlm.nih.gov/pmc/articles/PMC5682182/.

77   Amy Mackelden, "Kanye West Just Announced His New Album is Related to His Mother's Death," *Bazaar*, April 29, 2018, https://www.harpersbazaar.com/celebrity/latest/a20093405/how-did-donda-west-die-kanye-west/.
78   Bruce Beacham, MS, MD, et al., "Equestrian Cold Panniculitis in Women," *JAMA Dermatology*, September 1980, https://jamanetwork.com/journals/jamadermatology/article-abstract/541352.
79   adipose tissue: connective tissue in which fat is stored and which has the cells distended by droplets of fat (Merriam-Webster online), https://www.merriam-webster.com/dictionary/adipose%20tissue.
80   Olivia Jakiel, "Linda Evangelista Says She's 'Pleased to Have Settled' CoolSculpting Case After Fat-Freezing Trauma," *People*, July 19, 2022, https://people.com/style/linda-evangelista-settled-coolsculpting-case-after-fat-freezing-trauma.
81   Deidre McPhillips, "1 in 8 adults in the US has taken Ozempic or another GLP-1 drug, KFF survey finds." CNN, May 10, 2024, https://www.cnn.com/2024/05/10/health/ozempic-glp-1-survey-kff/index.html.
82   Tina S. Alster and Jason R. Lupton, "Nonablative cutaneous remodeling using radiofrequency devices," National Library of Medicine, 2007, 487–491, https://pubmed.ncbi.nlm.nih.gov/17870527/.
83   Ryan M. Greene and Jeremy B. Green, "Skin tightening technologies," National Library of Medicine, February 2014, 62–67, https://pubmed.ncbi.nlm.nih.gov/24488639/.
84   Anthony Youn, "Nonsurgical face lift," National Library of Medicine, May 2007, https://pubmed.ncbi.nlm.nih.gov/17440388/; author reply 1951–1951.
85   Erez Dayan et al., "The Use of Radiofrequency in Aesthetic Surgery," American Society of Plastic Surgeons, August 2020, https://journals.lww.com/prsgo/fulltext/2020/08000/the_use_of_radiofrequency_in_aesthetic_surgery.16.aspx.
86   Mukta Arali and Rashmi Ulli, "Kurcha Chikitsa – An Ayurvedic way of microneedling," *Journal of Ayurveda and Holistic Medicine (JAHM)*, Volume 8, Number 6, February 21, 2021, https://jahm.co.in/index.php/jahm/article/view/80.
87   Acupuncture, *Britannica*, Last updated August 14, 2024, accessed August 29, 2024, https://www.britannica.com/science/acupuncture.
88   "How Does Body Image Affect Mental Health?" Integris Health, May 26, 2022, https://integrishealth.org/resources/on-your-health/2022/may/how-does-body-image-affect-mental-health.
89   Kerry Heath, "Body Image: What It Is & How It Affects Mental Health," Choosing Therapy, March 7, 2024, https://www.choosingtherapy.com/body-image/.
90   How to Spot Skin Cancer, American Academy of Dermatology, https://assets.ctfassets.net/1ny4yoiyrqia/2j7YE9TiVWiGflNp0jGAHw/1896f4276649c3c2a336bb0182ea2f91/how-to-spot-skin-cancer-infographic.pdf.

www.ingramcontent.com/pod-product-compliance
Lightning Source LLC
Chambersburg PA
CBHW020541030426
42337CB00013B/930